THE NEW GUIDE TO
WOMEN'S
HEALTH

THE NEW GUIDE TO WOMEN'S HEALTH

TIGER BOOKS INTERNATIONAL
LONDON

A QUARTO BOOK

© Quarto Publishing Limited, 1985

This edition first published 1990 by
Tiger Books International PLC London

This book was designed and produced by
Quarto Publishing plc
The Old Brewery, 6 Blundell Street
London N7 9BH

ISBN 1-85501-062-3

Editors: Annabel McLaren, Liz Davies
Assistant Editor: Michelle Newton

Art Editor: Moira Clinch
Designers: Andy Luckhurst, Hilary Krag

Art Director: Alastair Campbell
Editorial Director: Jim Miles
Photography: Jennifer Beeston, David Birch,
John Hesseltine, Ian Howes
Illustrators: Paula Youens, Sally Launder,
David Miller, Anne Savage
Exercise and fitness consultant: Bronwyn Williams
Supplementary text: Maggie Daykin

The authors would like to thank the director of the Early Diagnostic Unit,
Elizabeth Garratt Anderson Hospital for Women, London: also the staff of
the American Women's Health Center in Washington, DC and London —
Elizabeth O. Davidson, RN, Deborah Jewell, RN Betty Lyons and Winifred
Grieg.

Filmset by QV Typesetting Ltd, London
Origination by Hong Kong Graphic Arts, Hong Kong
Printed in Hong Kong by Lee Fung Asco Printers Ltd.

Picture Credits

Contents

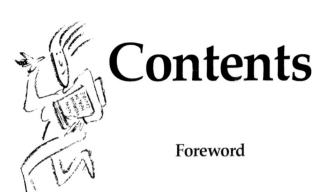

Foreword

Foreword

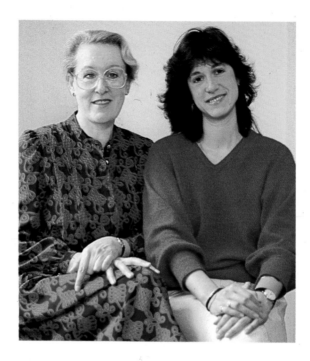

In the last decade, women in the Western world have become increasingly aware of the gap between the facilities provided for health care and their own actual health care needs. The crucial turning point is seen by many as the 1967 Abortion Act in the United Kingdom. Once women were given a choice in whether or not to receive ante-natal care or a termination of pregnancy, they realized that they could exercise choices in other aspects of their health care.

This book, which supports and encourages women's individual responsibility and choice, is a collaboration. One of us is a physician with over twenty year's experience in providing women's health care. The other is a writer who has specialized in the area of health, fitness and self-actualization for women. Though we belong to different generations — the one of us in her fifties and the other in her early thirties — we have found that our differences of experience have enriched our collaboration and, we hope, will be of benefit to you.

The issue of women's health is not the prerogative of doctors and medical specialists: our health cannot be separated from the other areas of our lives — work, sexual relationships, motherhood and so on. The physician may be the expert in contemporary medicine, but each individual patient is the expert on her own health and it is important for each woman to assess whatever medical care is advised with awareness and knowledge of her own body and her own life.

The increasing number of cases of early genital cancers in women is a cause for concern. There has also been an increase in sterility as a result of sexually transmitted diseases in women in their late twenties and early thirties. But the concept of early diagnosis and rapid, accurate treatment for sexually transmitted diseases — applying the knowledge gained from current research — may in the long run lead to a decrease in both serious pelvic infection and cancer.

Also, in the area of fertility, pre-conceptual care is becoming more and more of a reality. An awareness among women of the need to plan their motherhood as carefully as planning a career gives real meaning to the term 'family planning'. A very encouraging part of a gynaecologist's work nowadays involves teaching groups of women how to enhance their fertility and so get ready for a healthy pregnancy.

In the treatment of breast cancer it has been realized that many women have been mutilated unnecessarily — radical mastectomy could have been avoided had the women been taught and encouraged to perform simple self-examination and so discover abnormalities early on. Even now, the teaching of self-examination is not a regular part of women's health care in most family practices.

These factors indicate that women cannot simply leave their health care in the hands of the experts and specialists; consequently, self-help groups and co-operatives are growing fast — the most well-known being the Boston Women's Health Collective who produced the admirable women's health guide: Our Bodies, Ourselves. In the United Kingdom the Maternity Alliance was set up in 1981 by a group of women so that both professional health care workers and ordinary women could exchange information on the choices available in childbirth.

It has always been difficult to change a system from within and, until now, the male-orientated skills — like surgery — have been top of the hierarchy in medicine, while traditionally feminine ones, like nursing have been at the bottom.

This is now changing. The current rise in self-help and the ethic of care, primarily a move by women, for women, is a vital and optimistic development in promoting beneficial changes in the field of women's health care. Meanwhile, we can all play our part by looking to our own health, acquiring a basic working knowledge of our bodies, and applying that knowledge intelligently. It was to further this progress that we wrote this book.

Norma Williams

Hetty Einzig

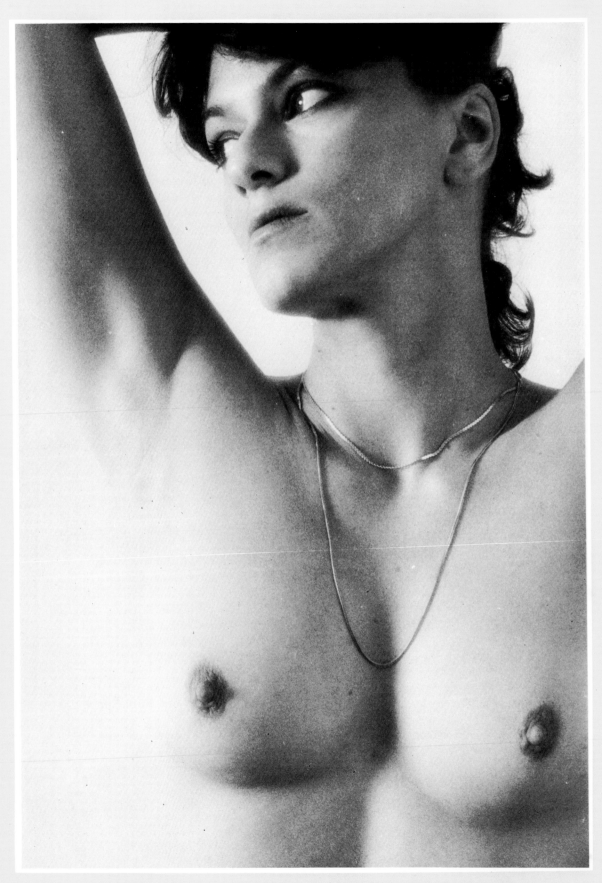

The Sexual Woman

The Female Anatomy · Hygiene · Self Discovery
Relationships and Expectations · Sexuality · Contraception
Sex and Society · Sexual and Physical Harassment · Rape

AS TODDLERS, BOTH GIRLS and boys take a great interest in their own and other children's genital areas. But by the time they are ready to go to playschool at three or four years old, most children have become aware from their parents' attitudes that such an interest is taboo, and this social conditioning is usually then reinforced at school. Such repression is now criticized by many progressive thinkers who believe that it may be responsible for sexual inhibitions in later life and, in the case of particularly sensitive or isolated children, may even make it difficult (or impossible) for them to form 'normal' sexual relationships when they become adult.

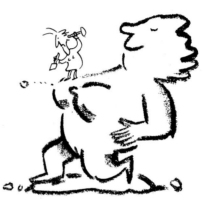

However, repressed or otherwise, most children fortunately do rediscover their sexuality in early adolescence. In girls this awareness often accompanies marked bodily changes — the development of breasts, and armpit and pubic hair — and the onset of menstruation as the release of the female hormones oestrogen and progesterone stimulate the reproductive system into activity

Most girls cope very well with these changes and even welcome them; but some find them slightly disturbing and even reject them, either developing personality problems or trying to return to their former figures by rigorous and increasingly obsessive dieting, culminating in the self-starvation illness called anorexia nervosa.

It is vitally important, therefore, that every young girl should receive timely and sensitive preparation for the onset of these changes which will enable her to develop into a self-confident and happy young woman.

The beginning of menstruation

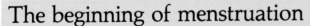

Most girls start menstruating somewhere between the ages of 11 and 15. The average age is 13, but some girls are ready physiologically — if not psychologically — to menstruate at nine or ten years old and some, although otherwise well developed, do not attain mature pelvic organs and regular menstruation until they are in their late teens. The onset of menstruation following any one of these patterns of development is perfectly normal; a girl's progress in development is quite often hereditary.

Several factors contribute to the timing of the onset of menstruation; among them height, weight and the nutritional standards of the family. Each woman has an individual range that is normal for her. And what is normal for her will change with each stage of her life: her menstrual cycle will both feel and be different when she is 30 from what it was at 15. This cyclical change in a woman's body continues until about her mid-forties or early fifties.

continued on p. 12

The female reproductive system

The female reproductive organs include the breasts, ovaries, Fallopian tubes, uterus and vagina. These organs have the capacity to produce and nurture a ripe egg, to nourish and house the growing fetus and also to provide food for the newborn infant and young baby. They *also control sexual response and the manufacture of the 'chemical messengers' called hormones, secreted by the endocrine glands.*

Hypothalamus: a collection of specialized nerve centres which control appetite, temperature and sleep, as well as secreting hormones — among them TSH, the thyroid stimulating hormone. In response to signals from the nervous system, the hypothalamus sends chemical 'releasing factors' to the pituitary gland.

Pituitary gland: the most important of the glands of the endocrine system, it controls the ovaries, the thyroid and the adrenal glands. It also secretes eight hormones. These include the 'gonadotrophins' FSH (follicle stimulating hormone) and LH (luteinizing hormone) which control sexual response and stimulate the production of oestrogen and progesterone, and oxytocin which triggers labour and causes the breasts to produce milk.

Thyroid gland: shaped like a butterfly, it sits directly over the windpipe; it controls growth and the metabolic rate — the speed at which oxygen and food are burnt to produce energy.

Adrenal glands: these make two vital hormones, adrenaline and noradrenaline, both produced when the brain senses danger.

Ovaries: these two glands produce eggs (ova) and hormones. With the onset of the menstrual cycle at puberty one egg is released every month and travels down one of the Fallopian tubes.

Breasts: the breasts contain milk glands, pectoral muscles, lymph nodes and fat. In early pregnancy the breasts enlarge, mainly through growth in the number and size of the glands. If a woman is breast feeding, the milk is stored below the nipple until some stimulus — a sucking baby, for example — causes it to be squirted out.

Fallopian tubes: these extend outward from the upper section of the uterus. Each tube is lined with tiny hairs which waft the egg towards the womb.

Vagina: a muscular passage leading at an angle from the vulva to the uterus. Its thick lining is composed of many folds of skin which enable it to enfold whatever is inserted — a penis, a tampon, or the woman's own fingers. Continual secretions keep the vagina healthy and moist.

The uterus, or womb, is a hollow, muscular organ. It consists of three parts: the corpus uteri (the body of the uterus), the isthmus (or neck) and the cervix uteri. The walls of the uterus are composed of muscle tissue. Within them lies the endometrium, in which the fertilized egg is implanted. If no egg is received the endometrium is shed as menstrual blood.

A woman's reproductive system is highly complex, designed as it is to convey a mature egg to a place where it can be fertilized by a male sperm.

The uterus, or womb, is the organ that protects the growing embryo for nine months — from conception to birth. The uterus is enclosed in a double layer of tissue.

Within this are the ovaries — the female sex glands, the equivalent of the male testes. They lie close to the openings of the Fallopian tubes and have two functions: the release of ova, or eggs, and the secretion of hormones. The view (right) shows the location of the female reproductive system in the lower abdomen.

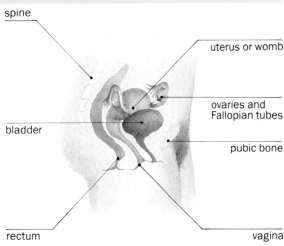

spine
uterus or womb
ovaries and Fallopian tubes
pubic bone
bladder
rectum
vagina

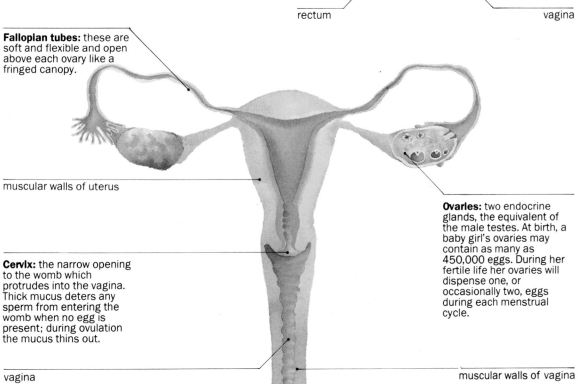

Fallopian tubes: these are soft and flexible and open above each ovary like a fringed canopy.

muscular walls of uterus

Cervix: the narrow opening to the womb which protrudes into the vagina. Thick mucus deters any sperm from entering the womb when no egg is present; during ovulation the mucus thins out.

vagina

Ovaries: two endocrine glands, the equivalent of the male testes. At birth, a baby girl's ovaries may contain as many as 450,000 eggs. During her fertile life her ovaries will dispense one, or occasionally two, eggs during each menstrual cycle.

muscular walls of vagina

A magnified cross-section through a Fallopian tube. Every woman normally has two of these tubes. Muscular contractions in the tube draw the egg, or ovum, into one or other of the tubes during alternate cycles. Halfway down the ovum hesitates for three or four days before being pushed rapidly into the uterus.

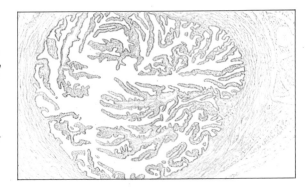

The menstrual cycle begins on the first day on which blood appears from the vagina, and lasts until the first day of the next period (bleeding). This cycle continually repeats itself until the onset of the menopause.

As well as physical responses to the cyclic hormonal changes, many women experience either mood elevation or premenstrual depression/tension. It is therefore useful for each woman to keep her own mood menstrual diary in order thus to develop an understanding of her own expected mental and physical changes during each cycle and gradually to evolve her own strategy for coping with them.

Other aspects of health and lifestyle can also affect the periods: whereas a period normally lasts anything between one and seven days (and should be considered abnormal if its duration is less or more than that), it is quite common for a woman's period to be delayed or even missed altogether as a result of stress, travel or illness.

Feminine hygiene

Each method of menstrual protection available today has its benefits and drawbacks, and only the individual woman can decide what feels comfortable and right. According to lifestyle a woman might choose tampons one month when expecting to be particularly active, and towels the next if that feels more comfortable. In the Third World most women keep a set of cloths for the purpose which are washed and re-used. At the other end of the spectrum some feminist centres in California offer the service of menstrual extraction, a gentle suction process which usually ensures that the whole period is over in as little as five minutes.

Your own comfort and a respect for your own body and its needs are the criteria for choosing sanitary protection, not the advertising claims for super-clean, deodorized products. Constant emphasis on the importance of ridding

A 'mood menstrual diary' enables every woman to know her own cycle, its effects on her moods and her response to the hormone changes that take place in her body.

There are women who experience the textbook 28 day cycle only interrupted by planned pregnancy: most of us, though, experience some degree of irregularity and discomfort which can cause unhappiness unless such feelings are understood and coped with.

The cycle begins on the first day of bleeding. Each day is divided into stages: morning, noon, afternoon, evening and night, because feelings in response to hormone change usually show a marked rhythm — some women experiencing depression and tension only at specific times of the day.

Moods are recorded by red ticks for heights of happiness, blue circles for calm efficiency, toleration and the ability to plan ahead. Black crosses denote

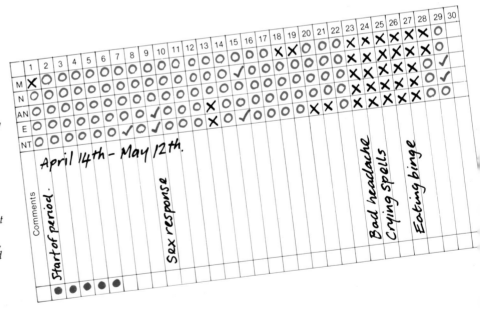

aggression, tearfulness and the loss of libido. It is important to record, once a day, the predominant feelings and emotions experienced in each stage of the day.

M morning	E evening	✓ heights of happiness
N noon	N night	O calm normality
AN afternoon		✗ depression/ bad temper

The events that take place during ovulation are quite dynamic: the ovum bursts through the ovarian wall and begins its journey down the Fallopian tube: if it does not meet a sperm it continues into the uterus and out with the menstrual flow.

At various points in the menstrual cycle the ovarian cells actually develop new structures — the follicles and the corpus luteum — as the ovary releases the egg and repairs itself. The illustration (below) shows the growth of the follicle that houses the developing ovum.

Just before ovulation a crop of follicles begins to develop, each of which consists of an egg surrounded by a layer of grainy cells. In the next couple of days about 20 of the follicles will continue to develop and enlarge. One or more of these follicles — now called secondary follicles — grows larger than the rest and bulges towards the outer surface of the ovary forming a bump. As ovulation approaches the ovary becomes enlarged with blood and the ligaments contract, pulling the ovary closer to the uterus. One of the follicles — now called the tertiary follicle — may grow to half the size of the ovary.

At the moment of ovulation the tertiary follicle wall ruptures and the egg (or ovum) oozes out. The burst follicle is now called the corpus luteum.

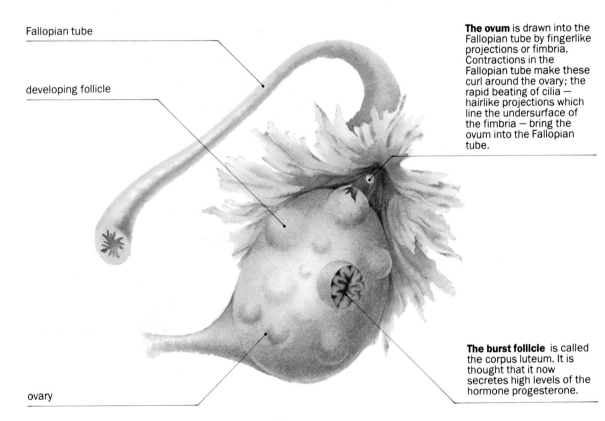

Fallopian tube

developing follicle

ovary

The ovum is drawn into the Fallopian tube by fingerlike projections or fimbria. Contractions in the Fallopian tube make these curl around the ovary; the rapid beating of cilia — hairlike projections which line the undersurface of the fimbria — bring the ovum into the Fallopian tube.

The burst follicle is called the corpus luteum. It is thought that it now secretes high levels of the hormone progesterone.

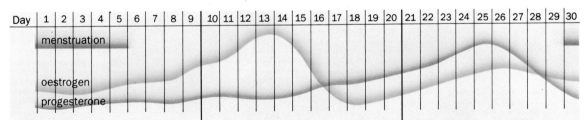

| Day | 1 | 2 | 3 | 4 | 5 | 6 | 7 | 8 | 9 | 10 | 11 | 12 | 13 | 14 | 15 | 16 | 17 | 18 | 19 | 20 | 21 | 22 | 23 | 24 | 25 | 26 | 27 | 28 | 29 | 30 |

menstruation

oestrogen

progesterone

The first phase: the first day of menstrual bleeding counts as day 1 and is usually a calm, happy time, although period pain may cause some discomfort. This phase of the cycle — leading up to ovulation — is characterized by the production of oestrogen — the 'happy hormone'.

The second phase: ovulation usually occurs around day 13 or 14, when oestrogen production is at its height. Many women can feel ovulation taking place; if they are planning to become pegnant making love during this time is obviously advisable.

The last phase: days 21 to 30 may be characterized by mood swings, depression and tearfulness. These feelings are usually put down to premenstrual tension (PMT) but they may well be explained as being 'post-ovulatory', when high levels of progesterone are secreted.

13

the body of any 'feminine odours' has led to the development of one or two products, the safety of which has been seriously questioned since the Toxic Shock Syndrome hit the headlines in the early 1980s.

This came about because many tampons are not subjected to the rigorous medical tests that are applied to surgical dressings. The use of synthetic materials instead of the traditional all-cotton fibres increased manufacturers' profits greatly but apparently contributed to high fever and debilitating infections in some women who bought the new tampons, which first came on to the market in 1978. They have since been withdrawn from the market.

Cleansing

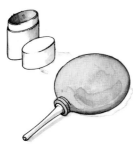

A small, French douching kit can be bought from chemists — it comes neatly packed inside a plastic container (above). Use tap water, flushing your vagina three times after sex. If the tap water is not safe, use bottled mineral water.

Keeping the genital area scrupulously clean by daily washing is obviously important in maintaining good health. All vaginal deodorants, sprays, perfumed bath oils, bubble baths and so on should, however, be avoided. These can cause severe irritation and inflammation, and may be responsible for many cases of recurrent cystitis and vaginitis. Cleansing of the vagina is nevertheless advisable.
- After menstruation.
- After sexual intercourse.
- For medical reasons such as changing the pH balance for the prevention of thrush (Candida albicans), or when taking antibiotics; for specific infections; during treatment for post-menopausal atrophic vaginitis; or after certain types of surgery.

Douching   Although not encouraged by medical practitioners, the process is very simple, and operates on the same basic principle as the genital cleansing jet of a bidet. Any sexually active woman is recommended to buy herself a douche-bag and learn to use it regularly. This helpful technique, which takes only a minute or so, can become just another good health habit like cleaning the teeth.

Self-discovery

Body awareness, which reaches a peak around the age of 13 or 14, is a vital part of self-discovery. It encompasses all aspects of your body: being aware of how you breathe, how you walk, how your breasts feel under your clothes, how your hair feels when combed, how your legs feel when they brush against one another. An adolescent also becomes acutely aware of the effect of her body on other people, even though she may not be able to verbalize her awareness, see also page 34. This self-discovery, self-knowledge and self-presentation are all part of being sexual.

Self-caressing, which begins at this time and continues throughout our lives, involves the gentle, usually unconscious but pleasurable, touching of one's own body in ways that are not obviously sexual: fingering an ear lobe for instance, prolonged hair brushing, smoothing body lotions and oils into our skin, manicuring our nails, making up, putting on stockings or tights. All these activities, even though some have clearly practical purposes, also involve us in touching ourselves in a sensitive way and thus contribute to our body awareness.

Our knowledge of the importance of caressing, whether by ourselves or others, was greatly increased by the work of the American gynaecologist Dr W.H. Masters and his wife and colleague, Virginia Johnson-Masters, who in their re-thinking of the nature of sexual response emphasized the importance of conditioning through 'sensate focus'. This is a technique by which couples who have experienced difficulties in relating to one another sexually, learn to respond to each other's bodies through non-erotic massage that slowly develops by gradual stages into a sexual contact, as and when both partners are ready.

The main criticism of the work of Masters and Johnson-Masters is that the

The external female sex organs are known collectively as the vulva. They surround the vagina and urethral openings and are the most sensitive part of a woman's body.

Clitoris: this contains the many sensitive nerve endings which make it the key to sexual arousal for most women.

Labia minora: these inner lips enclose the clitoris and contain sebaceous glands that help to provide protection for the vulva from urine, germs and menstrual blood.

Labia majora: the outer lips extend from the mons pubis to the perineum. From puberty they are covered on their outer surface with pubic hair.

Clitoral hood: this covers the clitoral glans and shaft. The clitoris swells during sexual excitement and retreats under this hood at the peak.

Urethra: this is the tube that extends from the bladder to the vulva. It carries urine from the body.

Vagina: this is a muscular passageway, about 8cm (3in) long, that extends from the vulva to the neck of the womb (cervix). It is a potential space that can enlarge to fit a penis during intercourse or a baby at childbirth.

The labia majora and minora *vary greatly in size and shape from woman to woman; while this variation may cause anxiety, particularly to teenage girls, there is no 'right' or 'wrong' size — both large and small are perfectly normal. It is a good idea for girls to get to know what their sexual organs look like by using a hand mirror to look at them; in this way they will see what is 'normal' for them.*

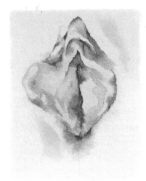 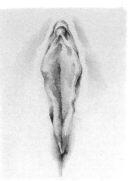

During a woman's sexually reproductive years, the labia majora are fatty and almost completely cover the external sex organs from view. The labia minora are relatively thin and delicate but during sexual arousal they swell and deepen in colour.

proposed therapy, by which individual couples are taught to re-explore and learn about each other's bodies and mental and physical responses, occurs naturally between couples — and it does not take a doctor to teach you to do what comes naturally.

The heightened physical awareness that comes with adolescence is often also accompanied by masturbation. For this usually solitary activity a girl may sit on the arm of a chair or a fence and rock back and forth to achieve clitoral stimulation. Or she may insert a finger into her vagina when in the bath, in bed or some other private place. Group activity in a summer camp or boarding school is also quite common. Shared by several girls, it is often innocently regarded simply as pleasurable fun. Two out of every three girls

Masturbation

15

PHEROMONES: YOUR NATURAL SCENT

A pheromone is a body odour which is special to each individual and which is picked up both by human beings and animals.

This natural 'scent' varies according to such factors as the stage reached in the menstrual cycle, pregnancy, stress, aggression and sexual attraction.

Perceptive women writers have noted the different odours of particular men: as far as Rebecca West was concerned, her lover H.G. Wells always 'smelt of honey', while Virginia Woolf claimed that, to her, a certain critic always smelt of 'stale meat'.

Anyone who has ever seen a mother with a new baby will notice how even the most meticulously made-up woman will touch her baby's head with her lips and, when encouraging her to breast-feed, will lick her forehead. This mutual exchange of tastes and smells is one of the reinforcements of bonding that takes place between a mother and her baby.

After examining a woman with a late period some practitioners are able to sense whether or not the pregnancy test will be positive; similarly, experienced midwives can often predict the length of a woman's labour from the chemical signals she gives out.

Our society has become highly conscious of body smells, perhaps because they act so instantly and powerfully on the subconscious. Women, in particular, are persuaded by advertisers to cover up their natural smells with heavy scents, under-arm deodorants and vaginal sprays. Unlike perfumes — which enhance your natural odour — deodorants are intended to mask the body's natural smell.

There are times during the menstrual cycle when a woman smells more 'sexy'

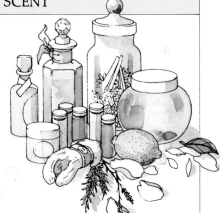

Perfumes are designed to work in harmony with the body's natural odour. Derived from the essential oils of plants, a perfume will never smell the same on any two people because each individual has their own body fragrance, dictated by their pheromones.

than at others — this often happens at ovulation. By keeping a menstrual diary a woman can be aware of when this occurs, and she can choose to enhance her own particular odour by wearing a favourite perfume.

masturbate by the time they are 16, and sociological surveys show that four out of five enjoy it.

Despite the many articles and sex manuals around today, however — all of which proclaim the naturalness of masturbation — some girls are still made to feel guilty about this perfectly normal activity and may grow up with a conviction that they are in some way disgusting or unclean, and may never have any intimate knowledge of their own bodies. Yet how can it be wrong or shameful for a girl or woman to touch a part of her body that eventually will be touched without embarrassment or shame by a lover, husband or male medical staff?

Masturbation is, and can remain, an intimate pleasure practised by many women throughout their lives — whether or not they have a partner. As Woody Allen remarked: 'The greatest thing about masturbation is that you don't have to dress up for it.'

Masturbation can also be an excellent treatment for spasmodic period pains. If you have moderately severe second-day pains, orgasmic response brought about through masturbation (or sex) can promote pelvic blood flow, and usually within 20 minutes the pain is much diminished. Many women who have not responded to any of the standard medical treatments for menstrual cramps have been greatly helped by this easy self-treatment.

Using a vibrator

Vibrators are sold in chemists, sex shops and by mail order, and are commonly used for self-stimulation, but it takes a little practice to learn to use one satisfactorily. The best way is to first place the vibrator against the underside of the clitoris and carefully, gently, stimulate the nerve endings. Be patient and do not expect an immediate response. Wait until you do begin to have a pleasurable response before actually inserting the vibrator into the vagina. It may help the first few times to lubricate the vaginal area with a little KY jelly. And just as with intercourse, using a vibrator is more comfortable with an empty bladder.

For a woman — even a woman who has a partner — who has never experienced an orgasm, experimenting in private with a vibrator is a good way to get rid of any inhibitions that may have been holding her back from discovering what kind of stimulation pleases her best. She should choose a time when she knows she will not be disturbed and take the time to find out if, for instance, she simply needs longer stimulation than she has ever previously enjoyed. (Some women can achieve an orgasm in a few minutes, whereas others may take up to an hour.) And once she knows what turns her on, she should not hesitate to let her partner know. Mutual satisfaction can only make sexual experiences more pleasurable for both.

Lesbianism

Women working together in small groups are often very aware of each other as individuals. Particularly in situations where, as a group, they are under stress — for instance, night-nurses in intensive care units, or women police officers in a receiving centre — very strong friendships and both mental and physical bonding can occur. Throughout history women have lived together as couples; more recently, lesbians as a social group have openly declared themselves and are now also able to fulfil their needs as mothers.

In retrospect many of us can remember women teachers at school who seemed different from other female staff, or who may have been living together and were the subject of gossip accompanied by nervous giggles and a mixture of fascination and derision for their sexual choice. We tend to stigmatize things that threaten us or do not conform to our idea of conventional behaviour, and lesbianism, like male homosexuality, may disturb our sense of the 'usual'.

In fact, lesbianism is still considered by some to be more abnormal than male homosexuality, and therefore harder to accept, largely because the tradition of male homosexuality goes back even further than the ancient Greeks and has accordingly received much attention in art and literature. Apart from the occasional isolated figure, lesbians have on the other hand only recently begun to find their voice. The fact is, however, that unless there is chromosomal abnormality, lesbianism — in the same way as hetero-sexuality — depends on the choices women make as a result of life experiences. A woman who had a severely repressive father, for instance, or who has had several disastrous relationships with aggressively dominant male partners, may grow to prefer a gentler partner of her own sex. Or she may simply find she has more empathy with other women.

Most girls as they grow up experience physical relationships with other girls, perhaps exploring each other's bodies, dressing up and playing at mummies and daddies or doctors and patients, or staying overnight with a best friend and sharing her bed. This is a normal part of growing up and of self-discovery, a part of developing body awareness and female sexuality. Even after these early experiments, most women continue to form deep friendships, particularly in their early twenties, and before they marry and have a family. Again, this follows the instinctive need of women to gain love and support from their own kind in a world that has always been less than fair to the female sex.

Indeed, the very formation of female gender identity takes place in the context of a close relationship with the mother, whereas — after the intimacy of breast-feeding — male gender identity is formed through separation from the mother, who acknowledges the boy to be different from herself and encourages his male separateness. This early behavioural conditioning enables women to feel comfortable and safe in close relationships with either their own or the opposite sex, whereas men experience greater ease as separate, circumscribed individuals, and may even perceive intimate relationships as threats to their masculinity.

As long as the decision to love and partner another woman is a considered choice based on an understanding of one's own sexuality then there is nothing wrong with lesbianism. As far as a woman's health is concerned it is, in fact, far less hazardous than either male homosexuality or heterosexuality: reliable statistics about lesbians' health are not yet available, but women together are less likely to experience venereal disease or cancer of the cervix, for instance, and to date there is no lesbian disorder equivalent to the epidemic of AIDS (acquired immune deficiency syndrome — in which the body loses its resistance to infection and malignant disease) among the male homosexual population. The few women who have suffered this latter disease have done so through contact with male partners.

Coming out If you have lesbian tendencies, or feel that you might have but are uncertain, it will almost certainly help you to seek out a lesbian club in your area. If you live in a large city, the chances are that you will be able to contact one through the advertisement section of a local newspaper. Or you may already have a female or male homosexual acquaintance who could provide you with this information. If contact with committed lesbians convinces you that you wish to join their number, they will be able to advise you about the inevitable changes in lifestyle, and the stresses as well as the relief that flow from such a decision.

You may, for instance, be pressured into changing your job. Some employers are still rigidly set against employing homosexual staff, particularly in areas such as educational or social work, where your possibly 'undesirable' influence on young children will be seen as a negative factor. If you are a lesbian mother you may come under similar pressure, and the mothers of other children at your child's school or playgroup may regard you with suspicion or distaste. In these and like situations you will need all your courage and convictions to continue — and having lesbian friends can then stand you in good stead.

Relationships and expectations

Sexual activity means something different to every woman, and something different to the same woman at different times of her life. In general, however, sexual activity is not an end in itself for most women but an activity that takes place in the context of a relationship. Given that, it is worth taking a look at the expectations women today have of their partners and how they have changed in the past 50 years or so.

Following World War I, the numbers of men of marriageable age decreased sharply, but even in times of peace, the mortality rate of young men between the ages of 15 and 25 is twelve times that of women of the same age — so there are never as many men as there are women as potential partners when it comes to marriage and starting a family. Society adapts to this fact and every decade has seen radical and rapid changes in the expectations and behaviour of women. In the 1920s flappers reacted to the wartime decimation of young men by wearing the bustless dress and consoling themselves by having a good time. In the 1930s, and the Depression, the marriage rate went up slightly but women married later and fertility rates decreased. The concept of marriage as an ideal, permanent state was interrupted again by World War II and following this came the 'baby boom'. Hearth and home were resurrected as an ideal in the 1950s and once again people married younger.

With the advent of oral contraception in the 1960s, it became generally acceptable for young people to have pre-marital sex and multiple partners.

The 1970s saw rising divorce rates and now, in the 1980s, more and more women who would like a permanent relationship find that, through education and work opportunities their expectations have risen and men of equal educational attainment and lifestyle are more difficult to find. Women are increasingly choosing their partners from a wider range of men, rather than following the once traditional pattern of marrying within their own social scale. Also, more and more women are getting married and having children without any longer having the deep belief that marriage is a permanent state. The idea of being faithful to one person for only a certain length of time, or 'sequential marriage' as the film star, Elizabeth Taylor, puts it, has taken root.

What is sex?

At its most fundamental, sex is nature's way of ensuring the continuation of the human race. But because we are complex beings with emotional needs, sex is also the physical means by which we cement relationships. This was not always so. In earlier times sex was often brutish, short and, for the majority of women, something which was done to them rather than an act of love in which they participated. It was only gradually towards the end of the eighteenth century, as health improved and as women's status slowly began to rise, that sense and sensibility were cultivated, bringing tender emotions into sexual relationships.

But for women it was not until the advent of widely-available contraception that sex could begin to be separated from procreation, or indeed could a more romantic and profound view of the sexual act be realized. Sex has now come to mean the contact with and relationship with another human being on the most intimate level, and we experience sex — at its best — as a physical communion between two people, to be valued as a basically happy and enriching experience, which adds to our sense of well-being.

Adolescent girls often have their first sexual experience through sheer curiosity, then wonder why it does nothing for them, what all the fuss is about, why they feel so uncomfortable or anxious. For many women, a first sexual encounter with a man is likely to be unsatisfactory. Many report that

First sexual experience

PHASES OF A SEXUAL RELATIONSHIP

Despite the changes in expectation outlined in the previous section, the phases of sexual activity remain much the same as in earlier days.

When you are attracted to someone, you instinctively organize your life so that you can have the maximum opportunity to get to know one another: plenty of eye contact, verbal contact and non-erotic physical contact. This phase used to be called courtship, when timid smiles were exchanged and men brought flowers and 'walked out' with their sweethearts.

If the relationship progresses to mutual satisfaction, erotic contact begins; this is whatever it means to each woman short of actually sleeping together, and having intercourse.

If erotic contact is mutually satisfactory, then the partners progress to the full sexual experience.

The whole process varies according to each woman and her partner, and may last for a period of time as short as a few hours or take a number of years — depending on background, inclinations and personal rhythms.

Post-coital tristesse is the term given to the lingering feeling of sadness that women occasionally experience after a sexual encounter. Such negative emotions are more likely to occur after chance liasons, but some women do report these findings in long-term relationships.

The process of learning from mistakes plus greater awareness and self-confidence should, in time, give these women the inner strength to cope with such emotions, making their experience of their own sexuality more positive.

theirs was a total disaster. Sex is likely to be mutually satisfactory only after both partners have got to know each other physically and can relax and trust each other.

Different rhythms   A major factor is the very different arousal patterns of men and women, in which men are aroused, peak and are satisfied quickly, whereas women take much longer to be aroused, stay at a high plateau for longer and take longer to reach an orgasm.

Because of these fundamentally divergent rhythms, sexual harmony between men and women is not automatic and natural. Human sexuality, bound up with emotions, social customs, fears and physiological differences, is complex and, to a great extent, a learned skill. This does not mean, however, that everyone does, or should, need to read a sex manual to learn how to make love. Good, mutually satisfactory sex, which both men and women should expect as their right, does not always happen 'naturally', but can be learned, as a child learns to walk and talk, through repetition, experience, trial and error, either with one partner or several. This learning process continues throughout life.

Tightness of the vagina   Some girls and women experience difficulty or discomfort in their first sexual encounter due to tightness of the vagina, either just around the opening or deep inside the vagina. This can be due to tension of the muscles (through nervousness or anxiety) or simply because the vagina has never been penetrated by a penis before. In either case, a woman can help herself by gently inserting first one, then two or three fingers into her vagina in the relaxing privacy of her bedroom or bathroom. In this way she can learn how her pelvic muscles work and how to control them.

The female pelvis   Many women have little or no idea of the anatomy and physiology of their pelvis; consequently the sexual act is something which they feel they have no control over. Yet being an active participant is essential for satisfactory sex.

To familiarize yourself with your own body, a useful thing to do, when

The male body is in a state of constant sexual readiness. The sperm that fertilizes the female ovum is prepared and stored throughout a man's sexually active life. A woman should learn about her partner's sex organs in order to achieve mutually satisfactory lovemaking and to understand how certain contraceptive measures, such as the condom and the cervical cap, can prevent fertilization.

The vas deferens are tubes that carry the developing sperm to the prostate gland. They are cut during a vasectomy.

The urethra carries semen to the penis and urine from the bladder.

The penis is composed of spongy tissue that becomes erect during sexual excitement, ejecting seminal fluid through the opening at its tip during orgasm.

The seminal vesicles make seminal fluid to supplement that made by the prostate.

The prostate gland produces seminal fluid that combines with the maturing sperm to produce semen.

The epididymis are connected to each testis by a small tube; they store and develop the sperm that the testes produce.

The testes lie within the scrotum and have a similar role to the female ovaries: they produce hundreds of millions of sperm cells daily, plus the male sex hormone, testosterone.

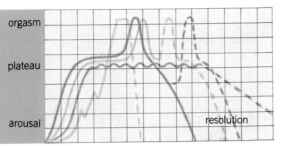

Patterns of female sexual response vary from one woman to another; the varying range of female response is suggested in red/yellow/orange (right). Male sexual response is less varied, and is indicated in blue.

orgasm
plateau
arousal
resolution

Orgasm: *this feeling of sheer pleasure originating in the pelvis, spreading throughout the body, is different for every individual. It can take longer to achieve for some and it is vital that a woman lets her partner know what gives her pleasure.*

Male and female sexual responses differ in that men are more quick to come to a peak of sexual excitement than women, whose sexual response is more complex. The researchers Masters and Masters-Johnson have divided the female sexual response into four phases.

Excitement or arousal: *in women this tends to result from physical contact rather than from visual stimuli and can also relate to the time in the menstrual cycle. During this phase the nipples become erect, the lips surrounding the vagina become swollen with blood and secretions* increase within the vagina.

Plateau: *the vagina is lubricated and ready to receive the man's penis. Stimulation of her clitoris by her partner's fingers, tongue or penis should result in orgasm.*

Resolution: *this phase follows the contractions of the orgasm and a feeling of peace and tranquillity usually ensues as the tissues of the vulva and vagina gradually lose their increased blood supply.*

Normal genitalia

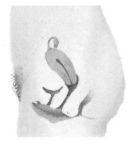

Genitalia during sexual response

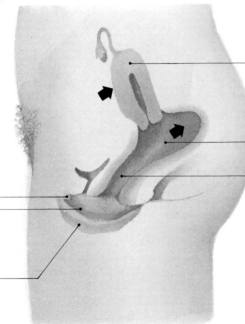

The uterus leaves its resting position during the plateau phase and rapidly descends again after orgasm.

The vagina increases in length and width in the plateau phase.

The contractions of the orgasm are localized around the lower part of the vagina, near to the opening.

The clitoris retracts during orgasm, though it may retract and re-emerge several times.

The labia minora expand markedly and protrude through the outer lips.

The labia majora open out slightly as a result of the increase in size of the inner lips.

urinating, is to stop the stream of urine and insert a finger into the vagina underneath the urethra — the opening to the bladder — and feel how tense the muscles are when contracted. Then slowly relax the pelvic muscles so that the flow of urine continues, over your hand, and you will feel how soft the pelvic muscles become. Don't worry about getting your hand covered in urine; simply wash your hand thoroughly afterwards. Continue this practice until you are familiar with the way your pelvis works. Once you have learnt to control these muscles so that you can relax or tighten them at will, your sexual experience — and that of your partner — will become much more pleasurable.

Many couples begin by having sex in the so-called 'missionary' position, with the man on top. This is the most widely practised position and the one in which each partner may feel most confident. However, there are many other positions which give both pleasure and variety, or greater comfort in such

Extending sexual experience

LOVEMAKING

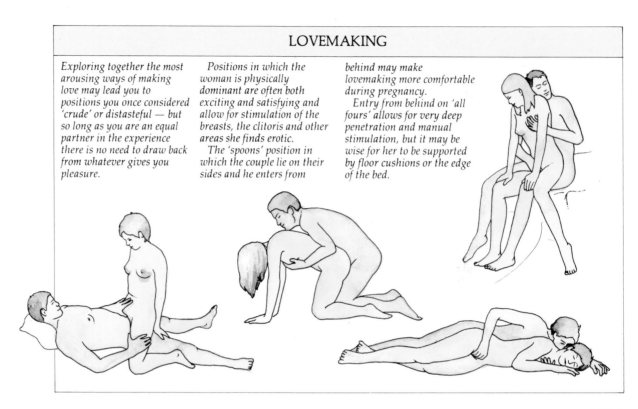

Exploring together the most arousing ways of making love may lead you to positions you once considered 'crude' or distasteful — but so long as you are an equal partner in the experience there is no need to draw back from whatever gives you pleasure.

Positions in which the woman is physically dominant are often both exciting and satisfying and allow for stimulation of the breasts, the clitoris and other areas she finds erotic.

The 'spoons' position in which the couple lie on their sides and he enters from

behind may make lovemaking more comfortable during pregnancy.

Entry from behind on 'all fours' allows for very deep penetration and manual stimulation, but it may be wise for her to be supported by floor cushions or the edge of the bed.

times as towards the end of pregnancy, when the woman's distended stomach prohibits the 'missionary' position, or when the man is substantially heavier than his partner.

Oral sex Both cunnilingus (in which the man has mouth and tongue contact with a woman's vagina) and fellatio (where the woman takes the penis in her mouth), are entirely matters of personal choice. Nowadays, oral sex has become widely accepted, and in consequence a lot of people have come to feel inadequate or old fashioned if they do not indulge. There is no 'must' about oral sex. Some women enjoy it, some do not.

As for sexually transmitted diseases and other complications, an infection is no more likely to come through oral sex but, as with all sexual contact, it is sensible to follow proper washing procedures for the vagina, penis, hands and mouth beforehand. Even so, in some women, the normal vaginal germs may be disturbed, possibly causing irritation. Also, just as with vaginal sex, skill at oral sex is not automatic; it takes time, patience and trust to learn. On a cautionary note, it should never be practised when either partner has a cold sore (herpes simplex) on their mouth.

Anal sex The case for anal sex is less simple. Firstly, it is usually extremely uncomfortable for women, sometimes causing ruptures and bleeding. Secondly, the rectum harbours bacteria which, as long as they stay there are harmless, but if they are transmitted elsewhere can cause serious problems. Two in particular — *Escherichia coli* and one of the genus *Haemophilus* — are major culprits in many vaginal and bladder infections. The penis should *never* be inserted into the vagina or mouth after anal sex, and should be thoroughly cleaned before sexual contact is resumed.

Again, anal sex is a matter of personal choice, although the risk of infection both for women and men is increased. No woman should feel that she 'ought' to indulge in this sexual activity, and she should resist the pressures of her partner, of fashion, or peer group one-upmanship which might make her go against her better judgement as to what feels right for her.

Sex therapy

If you and your partner feel that you have a sexual problem which you cannot resolve then your doctor or family planning clinic may suggest a programme of sex therapy where you will be encouraged to think positively and to learn to explore your sexual responses free from anxiety about 'performance'.

One of the problems about heterosexual intercourse is that the timing of sexual response, although extremely varied for each individual, usually shows a marked difference in rhythm between men and women. A man is easily aroused by visual signals, whereas a woman usually needs a feeling of safety, pheromone compatibility, see page 16, and the building of a gradual response to sexual intimacy that can vary from less than a minute to longer than an hour and a half.

The majority of men who can sustain an erection will usually ejaculate, but for many women orgasmic response only occurs around 50 per cent of the time. One of the most frequently-voiced psychosexual complaints from women is that of inability to achieve orgasm; indeed, this is like mathematical or musical ability: there is an enormous amount of variation and while some women are good at orgasmic response — they have 'perfect pitch' as it were — many others do need to learn how to reach orgasm.

The different responses of men and women, once they are understood, can be a source of mutual pleasure and mutual variation. Working on a turn and turn about basis — an approach often suggested by the therapist — to achieve mutual response is often extremely rewarding.

MYTHS ABOUT SEX

How long should sex last?
According to an academic expert in human sexuality, many Western men can sustain sexual intercourse for just a few minutes, whereas many women require at least ten minutes', or longer, physical stimulation to reach orgasmic response. The pattern of most couple's sex play therefore generally includes some manual stimulation before penetration. Some women are very pleased if men come quickly once they have penetrated the vagina; this makes them feel sexually powerful. Other women feel cheated if the man is exhausted after an orgasm and cannot indulge in further sexual stimulation. This is another situation when the use of a vibrator may be an acceptable solution for both partners. However, just as every sexual encounter is an individual affair, so there are no norms for the duration of intercourse and it is important that no woman lets her personal response be coloured by myths she may have absorbed about 'good' sex lasting for 'hours'.

Mutual orgasmic response
Climaxing together is often thought to be the height and aim of all sexual pleasure. All the same, it is a rare occurrence and not necessarily better or worse for each partner than experiencing an orgasm separately. Indeed, some women feel that their own orgasm becomes somehow 'submerged' if the man climaxes at the same time. The most usual orgasmic pattern is the man climaxing first and the woman climaxing some time afterwards, but again this depends on a host of factors, and many men delay their orgasm until the woman reaches a peak of sensation.

Size of vagina or penis Myth has it that large penises and slim, tight vaginas are best. This myth is harmful in that it puts a simplistic emphasis on sexual organs as status symbols rather than as parts of a whole sexual relationship and response. Vaginas have the elasticity and muscular construction to adapt to all sizes of penis and it is rare for women to complain that a penis is not large enough. However some women, after the birth of their first child, do find that their partner's penis feels too small. But as the vagina becomes toned again the problem is usually allayed.

Multiple orgasms Another myth which has caused doubts and anxiety among women is that of multiple orgasms. Sex is different for every individual, and so are orgasms. Some women experience frequent shallow orgasmic contractions, other women have one, deep uterine orgasm. An individual's orgasmic pattern changes throughout life, however, and as long as a woman truly feels sexually fulfilled there is no special merit in any particular orgasmic response.

Contraception

We now have a wide choice of contraceptives, yet they are still used by only about a third of all women during their fertile years, for reasons as varied as the choices available. In some countries modern contraceptives are not very well known; in others they are illegal, and even where they are not, social or religious pressures can make it difficult for women to control their own fertility as they may wish.

In contrast, countries struggling to control too rapid a population growth restrict the number of children a couple may have, and that limit may be one only. So, even today, many of the world's women have little or no choice in this fundamental role of procreation. All the more reason then, that those of us who do have the choice should know all the available options, what considerations apply to each of them and, particularly, the most up-to-date information on possible side-effects and long-term risks. Then we can exercise the prerogative of choice according to our individual priorities: health, age, lifestyle and so on.

Contraception is any technique or means used to control natural reproduction and, according to which one is used, there are several possible 'control stages' in the reproductive cycle. Again, according to the method used, either you or your partner may be solely responsible. You may choose to use a traditional means of contraception such as relying on lowered fertility during lactation (breast-feeding) or practising withdrawal (coitus interruptus) during intercourse; or you may use several different methods at different times, or in combination, and share the responsibility. But once conception has occurred, only you — the female partner — can do anything effective; if you decide on an abortion, however sure you may be that the pregnancy must be terminated, you may suffer intense psychological reactions later. Clearly, therefore, it is in your own best interests to use an efficient form of contraception until you are ready, if ever, to have a child and accept the great responsibilities as well as the rewards that this entails. Below, and on the following pages, you will find the information you need.

Natural methods

There are three methods of birth control that depend on the menstrual cycle's natural rhythm, and they can be used individually or in combination. As menstrual cycles cannot be relied upon to be entirely consistent, a combination of these methods is obviously likely to be more reliable than any one used in isolation.

Calendar

This entails keeping a day-by-day record of your cycle for eight consecutive months, noting the onset of bleeding as day one and the last day before your next menstrual bleeding as the final day of your cycle. This eight-month record will then show you your shortest and longest cycles — from which you can calculate your fertile days (see opposite).

Temperature

This involves taking your temperature, preferably using a basal body thermometer (which shows just the degrees 95 to 100, and has a mark for each tenth of a degree), every morning before you get out of bed — and before you reach for a cigarette or have a drink. The timing is very important, so don't wait until after you are up and dressed. Record the temperature on a chart the moment you have taken it.

As you keep these records, you will find that your temperature drops slightly 24 hours before ovulation, then rises to about half a degree higher than normal and remains thus for up to three days. During these four days you should not have intercourse if relying on this method of contraception. But as you also have to allow for the life-span of any sperm possibly present from previous intercourse, it is not a very efficient contraceptive method unless combined with the calendar and mucus methods.

CALCULATING YOUR FERTILE PERIOD

The first day of menstrual bleeding (day 1 of your period) counts as the first day of your cycle. Approximately 12 to 16 days before the start of your period (your next cycle) an egg will be released by one of your ovaries. While the egg lives for only around 24 hours, sperm can survive for up to 3 days — possibly longer. Because there is the chance of a variation of up to 5 days in the exact timing of ovulation, to calculate your fertile period you should add together:

- 1 day for ovulation.
- 4 days for possible survival of sperm.
- 5 days for variation in time of ovulation.

This gives you a total of 10 days when you may be fertile.

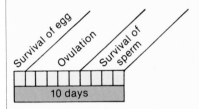

MONTH	APRIL / MAY

Chart — recorded fertility data:

DATE	16	17	18	19	20	21	22	23	24	25	26	27	28	29	30	1	2	3	4	5	6	7	8	9	10	11	12	13	14	15	16
DAY OF WEEK	T	W	T	F	S	S	M	T	W	T	F	S	S	M	T	W	T	F	S	S	M	T	W	T	F	S	S	M	T	W	T
DAY OF CYCLE	1	2	3	4	5	6	7	8	9	10	11	12	13	14	15	16	17	18	19	20	21	22	23	24	25	26	27	28	29	30	31	32	33	34

FERTILE PERIOD: shaded from day 15 to day 24.

SEX: X marks on various days.

MUCUS descriptions (Descriptive words such as: white, clear, creamy, wet, sticky, stringy, milky, cloudy, bloody, stiff, translucent): period, period, period, period, period, period, period, dry, dry, white cream, dry, dry, dry, dry, dry, tacky white, pasty white, pasty white, creamy white, wet and white, wet clear free-flowing, wet lots!, wet less, pasty scant, dry, dry, dry, tacky white, dry, dry, creamy white, dry, dry

Variations in your cycle

It is important that you keep detailed records of your cycles for at least 8 consecutive cycles before you embark on any of the natural methods of contraception. Even a very regular cycle may be disrupted by illness, stress or over-tiredness. Allowance for such variations needs to be taken into account when calculating your own safety margin; this allowance usually extends the 'fertile' period beyond the basic 10 days by another 2 or 3 days. Therefore:

- to determine the first unsafe day in your average cycle, subtract 18 from the number of days in your shortest cycle.
- to determine the last unsafe day in your average cycle, subtract 11 from the number of days in your longest cycle.

The following example assumes that your shortest cycle was 26 days and the longest was 31:

- first fertile day 26 minus 18 = day 8.
- last fertile day 31 minus 11 = day 20.

Therefore, taking the first day of your last period as day 1, you should consider yourself fertile from day 8 to day 20. These days are unsafe for intercourse and you should use some other method of contraception during the fertile period.

Longest cycle

1	2	3	4	5	6	7	8	9	10	11	12	13	14	15	16	17	18	19	20	21	22	23	24	25	26	27	28	29	30	31

11 days

Shortest cycle

1	2	3	4	5	6	7	8	9	10	11	12	13	14	15	16	17	18	19	20	21	22	23	24	25	26

18 days

Unsafe time

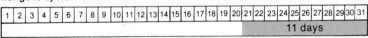

1	2	3	4	5	6	7	8	9	10	11	12	13	14	15	16	17	18	19	20	21	22	23	24	25	26	27	28	29	30	31

Unsafe time

25

Cervical mucus

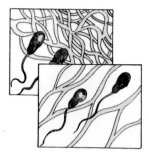

If you are observing your cervical mucus as a clue to ovulation you should check it first thing in the morning and a couple of times during the day, by inserting your forefinger into your vagina and noting its consistency in your menstrual diary.

During most of your cycle your mucus will be thick, possibly with a 'lattice work' pattern (above, top), forming a natural barrier to sperm. At ovulation it becomes free-flowing and slippery (above); when stretched between your fingers it forms strands. This mucus aids the passage of sperm, allowing them to swim up the vagina to the womb.

This involves becoming aware of the normal changes in the cervical secretions that occur throughout your cycle by inserting your forefinger into your vagina first thing in the morning — as with the temperature method, before peeing. You will notice that for a few days after menstrual bleeding, there is little secretion and consequently the vagina is quite dry; gradually, however, the secretion increases and becomes thicker, cloudy-white and sticky; as ovulation approaches, this secretion, or mucus, becomes clear, more liquid, slippery and stringy. If you insert a forefinger into your vagina at this time, this difference in the secretion is very evident. As soon as this change begins, and for three full days after, you should abstain from intercourse.

Advantages
- Apart from the initial cost of buying a thermometer for the temperature method, no other expense is involved in 'natural' methods.
- They are acceptable to certain religious groups.
- No medical risks are involved, with the exception of possible pregnancy if the method fails.

Disadvantages
- They seriously curtail freedom of lovemaking and consequently can cause stress for both partners.
- For many women who have irregular periods, it is complicated to calculate the 'safe' period. Some women have such irregular periods that a rhythm method is impossible.
- The temperature method may be rendered unreliable by illness.
- The mucus method can be misleading if sperm are also present.
- After a longish abstinence, the man may release older sperm in the course of ejaculation, and the woman may possibly still have within her an egg nearing the end of its fertility phase. If the sperm and egg should meet and fertilization take place, there is a risk of congenital abnormalities in the baby.
- If you and your partner are often apart due to work commitments, your limited time together could coincide with the fertile period.
- Intercourse may be robbed of spontaneity.

Barrier methods

Depending on which type is used, either partner can be responsible for birth-control by these contraceptives. They are as follows:

Diaphragms

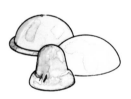

For many women, diaphragms and caps are the ideal method of contraception: there are few side-effects and, inserted properly, they give almost as good a level of contraceptive protection as the pill.

These shallow, dome-shaped rubber devices have a metal rim, also encased in rubber. The rim may be flat and compressible, or consist of a wire spiral. Either type fits over the cervix as a barrier against sperm trying to reach the womb and, as an added precaution, holds spermicide near the cervix.

Once spermicide has been applied to each side of the diaphragm and smeared evenly all over its surface and around the whole of the rim, it can be inserted at any time prior to sexual intercourse. But if this does not take place within two hours, you should insert additional spermicide into your vagina because the original application may no longer provide protection. Do not leave the diaphragm in indefinitely, but do leave it in place for at least six hours after intercourse; it will not interfere with urination.

Before you are fitted with a diaphragm, an internal examination is necessary because the doctor will need to determine the correct size for you. And as the vagina may change shape due to childbirth or substantial weight gain, for example, it is very important to have the fit checked every six months. In between times you should regularly examine the diaphragm because it can become thinner in patches due to wear. You should also replace your diaphragm every year.

Advantages
- It is almost as reliable as the pill, if used efficiently.

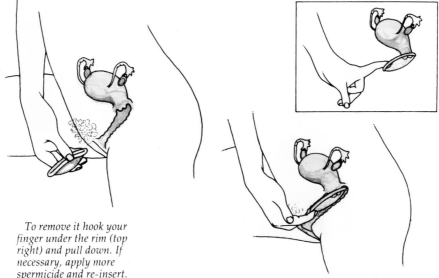

Wash your hands and apply spermicide to the diaphragm or, if you are practising, lubricate it with water or KY jelly.

Grasp the wire rim between your thumb and forefinger and push the diaphragm into your vagina towards your tailbone, just as you would insert a tampon. The diaphragm should flip neatly into place (far right) resting behind the pubic bone, covering the cervix (which feels like a solid lump) and fitting snugly into the posterior fold of the vagina.

Take a few steps around the room; if you can feel the diaphragm inside you it is either incorrectly inserted or it is the wrong size.

To remove it hook your finger under the rim (top right) and pull down. If necessary, apply more spermicide and re-insert.

- It does not cause any hormonal changes in your body.
- It is thought to help to limit the spread of vaginal infection and sexually transmitted diseases.

Disadvantages

A diaphragm may deteriorate unnoticed and become inefficient without warning for any of the following reasons:
- if kept in a warm damp atmosphere
- if the rim is bent out of shape
- if the rubber is damaged by your fingernails
- it will also be unreliable if it is not inserted correctly so that it covers your cervix completely.

Cervical caps

These are similar to a diaphragm, but smaller and less flexible. They can be shaped like a high-crowned hat with a brim, like a thimble, or a dome. But whatever the shape, the principle is the same: they all cover the cervix, are held in position by suction, and should be used in conjunction with a spermicide, according to the directions provided with them.

Women who have difficulty in retaining a diaphragm, and this is quite a common problem, may find these smaller caps a good alternative but, generally, the diaphragm is the more popular in Britain.

Condoms (sheaths)

This male contraceptive, made of latex rubber, is designed to cover the erect penis and to contain the ejaculated semen in its teat-like end. As the condom is smoothed onto the penis, the tip of the condom should be squeezed so that air cannot collect there. Generally, condoms are lubricated for ease of application over the erect penis and insertion into the vagina. They are available in various colours, some have ridges, which are supposed to enhance sensation for the woman, and some even have 'fingers and toes'.

Advantages
- Used efficiently, they are about as reliable as the diaphragm.
- They give some protection against sexually transmitted diseases.
- They are a good emergency contraceptive.
- As a condom, however fine and sensitive, dulls sensation slightly, this may assist the man in delaying orgasm until his partner is ready.
- Condoms are widely available and can be bought 'over the counter' from chemists and other shops.

Disadvantages
- They disrupt the spontaneity of sex.
- Lessen sensation for both partners.
- Can split, or be dislodged while the penis is still inside the vagina, spilling semen close to the cervix. (The detached condom is, however, easily removed from the vagina; it cannot be 'lost' there).
- Many women prefer to exercise personal control over their fertility.
- If condoms are carelessly stored, or more than a year old, they can deteriorate and therefore not give full protection.

Vaginal sponge

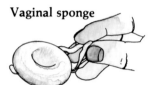

Vaginal sponges — which have recently come onto the market — were among the earliest of all contraceptive devices.

About 5cm (2in) thick and impregnated with spermicide, the vaginal sponge is concave on one side to fit over the cervix. The spermicide does not have to be 'topped up' so it is less messy than other barrier methods. It has to be kept in place for at least six hours after intercourse but can be left for up to 30 hours.

However, results from a recent clinical trial of sponge users (Margaret Pyke Centre, London 1984) has established that a high failure rate is associated with the sponge (25 out of 126 women becoming pregnant in a 12 month period); consequently it should only be used by women who do not mind if they become pregnant, or have a lowered fertility — perhaps because they are breast-feeding.

Spermicides

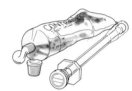

When used on their own spermicidal creams and foams should be inserted via an applicator which will ensure that the whole of the cervix is properly covered.

Spermicides come in the form of aerosol foams, foaming tablets, pessaries, creams, jellies and film and are widely available from chemists. Although some are intended to be used as the sole contraceptive medium, this is not really reliable even though they are designed to provide both a chemical and mechanical barrier against sperm entering the cervix. Preferably, they should be used with a diaphragm, cap or condom.

Advantages
- They do not alter your hormonal balance.
- They are easy to use.
- They provide extra lubrication.

Disadvantages
- Some people find them rather messy to use; at least, the creams and jellies.
- They can be disruptive to lovemaking as you must insert the spermicide at precisely the time recommended. You may also have difficulty in getting the timing right.

Intra-uterine devices (IUDs)

These plastic or copper devices are inserted into the womb and can be left there for a considerable time to make the womb hostile to implantation of a fertilized egg. They should, however, be changed every two or three years if made of copper. They come in a variety of shapes and sizes, but tend to be no longer than 3cm (1½in).

A pelvic examination is necessary, to enable the doctor to determine the size of IUD needed. This is then inserted into the womb with the aid of a hollow plastic tube, which is withdrawn leaving the IUD in place. A plastic string attached to the IUD is used to check that it has not been expelled, but the device should be removed by a qualified doctor, because if it is not removed correctly it can cause serious damage.

Advantages
- They are very reliable.
- They give long-term protection and are effective from the moment of insertion.
- They do not interfere with spontaneity or sensation during lovemaking and intercourse.
- They do not affect the body's natural hormone balance.

Disadvantages
● Most women experience some discomfort when they are first inserted, and some find this excessive.
● During insertion, perforation of the womb can sometimes occur.
● If you have an undetected vaginal infection at the time of the fitting, the device can carry it upwards into the womb. So if you experience some of the following:
● Discomfort on intercourse
● Changed or painful menstrual bleeding
● Discharge
● Bleeding
● Backache
Do check with you doctor or clinic. If you do have a vaginal infection it can be treated with antibiotics, but if it continues untreated it can spread to the Fallopian tubes and may even cause sterility. If you are experiencing any of these symptoms it is vital that you are examined: pelvic inflammatory disease (salpyngitis) can result, causing long-term ill health.
● When the device is first fitted, bleeding may occur on the first couple of days afterwards, and you may experience irregular bleeding between periods — which will tend to be heavier initially. In consequence you need to be on your guard against developing anaemia.
● Expulsion of the IUD can also occur, particularly in the first couple of months. As you may not even notice this, remember to check the string regularly as advised by the doctor or clinician.
● There is a higher risk of ectopic pregnancy.
● An IUD is most likely to cause side effects in young women and those who have not already had one or more children. It is sensible, therefore to postpone the use of an IUD until your family is complete.

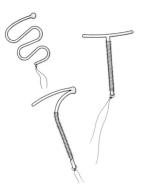

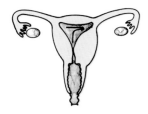

Left to right: the Lippes loop, the Copper 7 and the Copper T. IUDs are inserted into the womb (below) by means of a plunger or hollow tube; they act by making the womb hostile to the fertilized egg.

The pill contains synthetic oestrogen and progesterone — similar to the hormones naturally produced by the ovaries. However, the chemical versions alter the body's natural hormonal balance so that the ovaries do not release eggs as in a normal menstrual cycle. Because no eggs are released, the normal menstrual bleeding doesn't occur either, but there is some 'withdrawal bleeding', because the lining of the womb does still build up slightly. Depending on which pill is prescribed, a course is taken for either 21 or 28 consecutive days.

Today's pills have a much lower hormone content than the early forms and consequently the risks have been lessened; in fact if the low-dose combined pill contained much lower levels it would not be the reliable means of contraception it has proved itself to be over the last decade and a half.

The pill

Advantages
● Providing you take the pill correctly, it gives the best possible protection against an unwanted pregnancy, short of sterilization.
● It does not interfere with intercourse.
● Periods are predictable, even if previously you had irregular bleeding.

Disadvantages of the combined pill
● It can seriously affect your circulation, causing blood clots in the veins or arteries. This results in serious problems at any age but if you are over 35 it could be fatal.
● High blood pressure can also occur, particularly if you are overweight, or smoke. However, if you stop taking the pill, or change to the mini-pill, blood pressure usually returns to normal.
● Other possible side effects are: depression, nausea, dizzy spells and water retention. But most of these symptoms tend to disappear after your initial adjustment to taking the pill. If they do not, report the symptoms to your

doctor or clinician and consider changing to another pill with a different combination of the two hormones.

When not to take the pill   As the pill can only be prescribed by a family planning clinic or your doctor, usually you should be safeguarded by a routinely thorough check-up (including examination of your breasts, and a pap (cervical) smear). But just in case you do somehow 'slip through the system' you should be aware that it is not advisable for you to take the pill if you are over 35; if you are a heavy smoker; if you have a personal history or family history of heart disease and/or a clotting disorder.

Even if none of these factors are relevant to you, it is not advisable to stay on the pill indefinitely. Ideally, you should change to some other form of contraception after ten years. In the meantime, do have regular check-ups. And if you have any marked adverse reaction, do go to see your doctor about it — sooner rather than later.

Also, when you commence taking the pill, make sure that you clearly understand how long it will be before you are covered against the risk of conception, because this protection will not come into effect immediately.

If you miss a pill, but remember within 12 hours, take the one you missed straight away, and take the next one at the regular time. Even if it is longer than 12 hours before you remember, do the same, but you will also need to use an additional form of contraception for the next 14 days (do not stop taking the pill during this period).

If you are prescribed another drug, particularly an antibiotic while taking the pill, the contraceptive effectiveness of the latter may be lessened. To be on the safe side, use an additional method of contraception all the time you are taking the drug, and for 14 days afterwards. In fact, whenever you are prescribed a drug, it is good practice to check out with your doctor any possible side effects it may have, either alone or in combination with other drugs you may be taking — including the pill.

TYPES OF PILL

The 28-day pill is simply the ordinary combined pill supplemented by seven additional lactose pills of a different colour, included to allow continuity of daily intake so that you do not have to remember when to start taking the next course of pills again.

The mini-pill contains a lower dose of progesterone than most of the combined pills, and no oestrogen. For this reason, it only infrequently prevents release of an egg by either one of the ovaries. However, it does thicken the mucus present at the entrance to the cervix, and this makes it difficult for sperm to get through. Also,

there are normal periods, not 'withdrawal bleedings' as occur when taking the combined pill. The mini-pill has to be taken regularly, every morning without a break — even during menstrual bleeding.

Triphasic and biphasic pills are both variations of the combined pill, but the oestrogen and progesterone contents vary to accord with certain points in the cycle. Triphasic pills come in a three-colour pack, each colour having a different strength, and it is essential that you take them in correct sequence, according to the directions provided.

The newer biphasic pills must again be taken in the

correct sequence: the first seven in each course contain less progersterone than the remainder. But because these pills are relatively new, there has been less opportunity to study their possible long-term effects, so, if you are satisfied with the combined pill it is not advisable to change. But they may be helpful to women who experience problems with combined pills. It is beyond the scope of this book to give more detail, but your doctor or family planning clinic will probably be happy to provide more information.

At least 48 hours passes from the time when sperm meet the egg to the point when the fertilized egg bounces down the Fallopian tube (see page 112), and settles in the uterus. If, at this time either the hormonal balance of the physical structure of the endometrium (the tissue lining the uterus) is altered then implantation of the fertilized egg can be presented, and it will disintegrate, causing slightly less bleeding than is experienced in a normal period. There are a number of methods of post-coital contraception.

Morning after pill   These pills contain the same levels of hormones as four tablets of a moderately-dosed contraceptive pill (eg Eugynon 50). Two tablets should be taken as soon after intercourse as possible — certainly within 72 hours. The dose should then be repeated 12 hours later. Most doctors who prescribe this medication will ask you to tell them when your period begins.

IUD insertion   The insertion of an IUD within 24 hours of intercourse should prevent the implantation of the fertilized egg; this method, however, has a slightly higher failure rate than the morning after pill.

Menstrual extraction   A small plastic catheter is inserted through the vagina and into the uterus. The endometrium is drawn off either by means of a syringe or vacuum pump. This method is not available in the UK.

Vaginal suppository. Prostaglandin suppositories, placed in the vagina, have the effect of bringing on a period and emptying the uterus. They can be very useful, particularly when given in conjunction with a beta HGC blood test which can establish whether or not you are pregnant within 24 hours of intercourse.

This can be achieved in several ways, but the end result of all methods is to block the Fallopian tubes so that an egg cannot be fertilized. What actually happens is that each time an egg is released by one of the ovaries its normal progress along the tube is blocked and it dies there, eventually dissolving.

Some women may experience heavier periods after such an operation, but neither the menstrual cycle nor sex life are otherwise affected.

Advantages
- Sterilization is a highly effective form of birth control.
- There are usually no long-term side effects.

Disadvantages
- Occasionally, tubes have been known to rejoin. If this happens you will not know until, possibly, you become pregnant and an ectopic pregnancy can happen in such cases. Warning signs are a missed period and pains in the lower abdomen, followed by bleeding. See your doctor without delay if these symptoms occur.
- On the other hand, if the sterilization is 100 per cent effective and you later decide that you would like another child after all, you may deeply regret having undergone what is virtually an irreversible operation. So, if there is any possibility that you might have such second thoughts, you would be well advised to stay with one of the other forms of contraception.

Vasectomy is increasingly popular. It involves a simple 15 to 20 minute operation, under local anesthetic, to block off the vas deferens, see page 20, so that sperm cannot progress through the urethra and into the penis. This simply entails making two small cuts in the scrotum, one on each side, in order to reach the vas deferens tubes, which are each then 'tied off' in two places, and the portion of tube between each pair of ties is then removed, before the vas deferens are tucked back into the scrotum and the incisions stitched up.

Post-coital contraception

Sterilization
Female

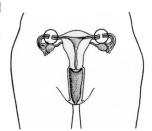

Tubal sterilization blocks both Fallopian tubes, thus preventing the sperm from meeting with the egg and fertilizing it. It does not stop egg manufacture in the ovaries. Because many women experience excessive bleeding after tubal litigation a careful history and full physical examination is essential before the procedure is carried out.

Male

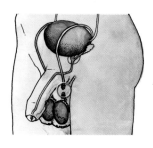

Vasectomy involves cutting the tubes (vas deferens) that carry the sperm from the testicles in the scrotum to the prostate gland. A fluid is still ejaculated during intercourse but it does not contain sperm.

Several follow-up tests are necessary to ensure that no sperm is present in the semen and until these tests are satisfactorily completed another form of contraception should be used.

Advantages
● Because the operation is so minor, the risk of complications is negligible.
● It is almost always 100 per cent effective (there have been well-publicized instances where a pregnancy has occurred after such 'sterilization').
● Sex drive is not affected and it does not affect hormone levels. Ejaculation occurs as usual, although there are no sperm present in the seminal fluid.

Disadvantages
● A vasectomy is virtually irreversible — so a man has to be certain that this is the correct course of action.
● Some discomfort may be felt for a few days after the surgical procedure has been carried out.

Social aspects of sex

Most couples starting out on married life make their wedding vows in all good faith, '...for richer, for poorer, in sickness and in health', but life has a way of constantly putting those vows to the test; how each couple faces up to such pressures can make or break the contract.

Today couples — young and old — and indeed, single people, are subjected to greater social pressures than ever before. In a time of still rising unemployment in many parts of the world, even those who have struggled their way through to a good, higher education have no guarantee of a job. We are now confronted with the social phenomenon of able-bodied, educated young people in their early twenties who have never had work experience, job satisfaction or the social independence that only a regular salary can bring.

Equally, age and experience are no shield against the great social dislocations which threaten everyone's well-being and happiness. Men and women who have worked for years in industry, building up skills and experience, are suddenly confronted by redundancy and early retirement; while some may welcome this opportunity to get off the treadmill of a routine job, others will find that such an unlooked-for change imposes intolerable strains on family relationships and marriage.

Young women who thought that having a baby would be the most romantic and fulfilling experience (or a pleasurable release from an un-fulfilling job with no prospects) may find themselves three or four years later trapped in a high-rise block of flats with two or more pre-school children and no hope of being rehoused or having enough money to buy even the basic necessities of life or to pay their mounting debts. Other women may struggle to maintain a balance between a stimulating job and being a wife and mother — perhaps coming under pressure to conform to the still widely-held ideal of motherhood while knowing, deep down, that caring for and bringing up children is not really an option they should have chosen. Such women — and their children — may be marked for many years by this conflict.

Many men are having to face up to the reality that if a wife's income is essential to maintaining a reasonable lifestyle, then standards in the care of the home can only be maintained if he undertakes a fair share of the load.

A man in the supermarket is no longer a rare sight — indeed he may be there because his wife has become the working partner while he, because of redundancy, illness, or role-reversal, has become the stay-at-home.

Unisex fashions and hairstyles have made their obvious contribution to changing attitudes towards male and female sexual stereotypes across the social spectrum. Even the advertisers are beginning to respond to increasing pressure from female consumers for more realistic portrayals of women — as a force to be reckoned with, rather than as mindless robots concerned mainly with biological stains or soft, smooth hands.

In short, sexual attitudes have undergone a great shaking up — and they show few signs of settling down even yet. Many of us are coping well, and even managing to raise an amused and indulgent smile at the more extreme alternative images that confront us on the small screen and in general media advertising. But by no means everyone responds well to these and other social stresses. In the following pages we deal with the three major sexually-orientated consequences of pressured lives that rebound on to women: incest, battering, and rape.

It has been estimated that in the Western world possibly one in 12 women have experienced incest. That is, sexual abuse or interference by a father, a brother or other male relative.

Incest happens right across the social classes, not just in deprived families. Sometimes the offender is a brother or an uncle, but most usually he is the father or stepfather. Sheila Kitzinger, a social anthropologist and childbirth educator, quotes studies which show that up to one quarter of the cases of incest occur with little girls under the age of five, and the victims are most likely to be around 10 or 11 years old. A.C. Kinsey (author of *The Kinsey Report*) found that 25 per cent of the white middle-class women in his study claimed to have had sexual relations as a child with an adult man. An American television programme, *The Last Taboo*, screened in 1979, received in response over 4,000 telephone calls. So, far from being something that happens to other people or in remote, primitive areas of the world, incest is prevalent and cannot be ignored in any consideration of how women experience their sexuality in society today.

The dividing line between incest and normal, affectionate, loving, physical contact within the family is very fine. Most girls go through two phases of being seductive as they become aware of and explore their sexuality: first, between three and five years old and then again between 13 and 17, at which time their sexuality becomes more connected with a sense of responsibility

Incest

SEEKING HELP: INCEST

Not all women are traumatized by such experiences and some have reported that the experience was not totally negative, but a majority do find that later in life the experience — which may have been buried deep in their subconscious — affects their relationships with lovers, husbands or children.

Any mother, therefore, who suspects that her current husband's or lover's interest in her child or children is not normal should seek help — and particularly if her present husband is not the natural father. The number of children battered or killed every year by a stepfather or their mother's live-in lover runs into

several hundreds.

If the woman is herself experiencing difficulties within the marriage or relationship she may be torn between a desire to salvage it and a deep instinctive urge to protect her children. If this is the case and she feels unable to approach a social worker for advice and assistance, then she should try to discuss her fears with her doctor. It may be possible to persuade the man in question to accept counselling or medical treatment.

Incest is a criminal offence and any woman who knowingly remains silent, whatever her reasons, is colluding in a serious crime against her child. Even the

most hardened criminals do not condone child molestation.

Any woman who feels guilty because she had such an experience in childhood should seek professional counselling. It will enable her to come to terms with the anger, grief, disgust, fear and other distressing emotions that underlie the guilt, and help her to put the experience into the context of her present life. Women have an innate tendency to feel that everything is their fault and to feel guilty, even about things that have been done to them by others, or about things over which they have no control.

33

and the social consequences of their behaviour. This seductiveness is a normal part of a girl's growing up — her way of testing what it is like to be a woman, and what effect she has on her parents and the people around her.

It is important for parents to be aware of this pattern in a girl's development and not to see her seductiveness as an invitation to molestation. Parents have a responsibility to behave as protective adults, providing a secure environment in which their child can feel able to take the risks involved in growing up and moving out into the world. Traditionally, the father is the parent who provides the bridge between the security of the home and the challenges of the outside world.

Conflicting emotions   In cases of incest in which the child is a substitute for a dead or absent mother, she is usually better able to cope with the situation than in other cases in which she is a 'rival' to her mother. In the latter situation the girl experiences a whole complex of conflicting emotions: fear of incurring her mother's wrath, guilt at deceiving her, possibly desire to replace her as the woman in her father's life, or loss of security and trust in her parents' desire and ability to protect, love and nurture her.

Sometimes a mother can unwittingly play a part in the occurrence of incest, either because she has herself rejected sexual relations with her husband, or uses her daughter as an object in power games with her husband: 'Just you wait till your father comes home!'

Everyone reacts emotionally to incest. But shock, horror, disgust and outrage are the most usual immediate responses and it is not uncommon for mothers to turn on their daughters and blame them for 'breaking up the family', causing tremendous guilt in the girl for the 'trouble she has caused'. This guilt can endure long into adult life, affecting all her future relationships.

Battered women

The incidence of non-accidental injury to children has been a recognized social problem since the late 1950s, but only in the last ten years or so has the reality of battered women come to light. The first refuge for battered wives in the UK was organized by Erin Pizzey in 1971; since then the phenomenon of the battered woman has been widely publicized and other centres have opened to provide refuge and a support system for the unfortunate victims of such domestic violence.

Although it is usually more obvious in lower social classes, the incidence of battering occurs at every level of society. Battering can range from extreme physical violence, resulting in injuries so severe that the victim may be hospitalized, to a more subtle but insidious psychological battering that leaves the woman convinced that she has little worth, no independence and is lucky to have attracted any man at all.

Why be a victim?   There is a curious, popular myth that many victims of battering actually enjoy the experience in a masochistic way, and stay with the batterer because they cannot imagine or cope with any other existence. Or it is supposed that since an argument 'takes two', the injured woman must have provoked such attack. Otherwise, goes the argument, why doesn't she simply leave her tormentor? The harsh fact is, of course, that many such women are in no position to leave, for a complex variety of reasons — economic, social and psychological. Perhaps most trapped of all is the woman with two, three or more children of under school-age who may also be subjected to violence. Indeed, the woman may have been ill-treated similarly by her own father while she was a child.

Profile of a batterer   The sort of man who inflicts such misery may be superficially charming, and educated, but is often also pathologically jealous. Such men are found in all walks of life; for instance, he may be an impotent businessman, a timid sales assistant or a macho lorry driver, each venting his usually concealed frustrations on home ground. He may actually suffer the same sense of low self-esteem as his partner and resort to displays of superior strength mainly to boost his own ego. Many such men also have very rigid and limited views about sexual roles: man as the dominant partner and woman as the stay-at-home wife, subservient, passive and bound to him by wifely duty. He may actually feel a sense of grievance that his partner leaves the burden of decision-making to him, yet at the same time make it all too plain that he will brook no 'interference' from her in major — or minor — issues.

Violence begets violence   Many such relationships may initially seem to be ideal matches, each partner subconsciously adopting a stereotyped, complementary sexual role. But, inevitably, there will be stresses too, and tension is likely to mount to the point where a first blow is struck, sincerely atoned for, forgiven and temporarily forgotten. But the next time it will be struck more

SEEKING HELP: BATTERED WOMEN

Men who, under the influence of sexual frustration or alcohol, can only release their vindictive, inadequate feelings by violence, can sometimes be changed by behavioural therapy. However, if the woman decides that her relationship is valuable enough to her and her partner for her to seek help, it is important that the 'contracting' necessary during this process is monitored by a professional group.

One of the good methods to have come out of the behavioural therapies recently is this concept of relationship contracting. For instance, during marriage counselling — after an initial interview during which each partner has discussed their problems from an individual point of view — the counsellor or therapist asks both partners to write down on a sheet of paper all the good points they can think of in relation to their partner, and on a second sheet all the bad points. After 10 to 15 minutes, first the good points and then the bad points are discussed.

The therapist then explains the concept of contracting — that of committing promises to writing, and trying to keep

them, is a reasonable and valid way of making a happier relationship. For instance, the mother of fairly young children may feel that she and her husband and children should all sit down to an evening meal together and may be very distressed if her husband consistently fails to come home in time to participate. The husband can promise that he will do his best to be home in time and if he cannot make it will telephone. In turn, the wife may promise not to nag or be reproachful when this occurs. After a period of about six weeks, the couple should bring back their daily 'action diaries' to discuss with the therapist.

It is important to realize that no points are won or lost, but that the action diaries must be strictly honest and relate only to factual events without any value judgements added. Also, because no human being can change more than one or two aspects of their behaviour at any one time, in order to achieve realistic results contracting should cover only one or two items of grievance in any six-week period. Contracting is a very useful way of clearing the decks for a more effective and

cooperative relationship.

If, however, the violence is such that the woman wishes only to escape it, there are organized shelters where she can find temporary refuge and support while she recovers sufficiently to make alternative arrangements. This temporary refuge may not always be particularly comfortable — indeed, it is quite likely to be crowded and afford little if any privacy — but she will be safe and she will be given help.

The Citizen's Advice Bureaux are good sources of advice about free legal aid, and legal protection is normally quickly available in the form of a court order restraining the husband or partner from further contact of any kind.

Any woman who has suffered serious injury as a result of battering should therefore present herself at the nearest hospital casualty department where, not only can she receive appropriate medical care, but she can place on record evidence of the degree of suffering inflicted upon her, evidence that the courts will give all due consideration.

easily, thereafter to be anticipated. Once a pattern of violence is thus established, it is very likely to escalate.

Rape

Rape can be defined as sexual penetration — or simply sexual contact — by a man against a woman's wishes. The majority of rapes are perpetrated by a man known to the woman, and often by a man within her close family or social circle. Many such attacks go unreported and the woman does not seek legal or medical help, either because she is too afraid or too embarrassed.

Although there are a few women who can come to terms with what has happened to them fairly quickly, can have a check-up, discuss the experience with a doctor or a close, trusted friend, and then put it firmly behind them — glad to have survived without any lasting physical damage — most women are mentally, if not physically, scarred. They experience a reaction of profound grief at this assault on their previously intact female gender identity and need to work through the resulting state of distress with sensitive, professional counselling. Gender identity is, after all, not simply a matter of knowing whether you are female or male, but more specifically having a strong sense of identity within a secure enviroment.

The sudden, violent act of rape violates a woman's sense of security, making her feel like a helpless object and violently shattering her self-esteem. Some women go into a state of mental shock; numbness, loss of memory, inability to speak or to show any emotion at all are just some of the extreme reactions. There is a feeling that 'If someone can do this to me then I must be nobody and nothing'. The pain of this feeling is often too great to bear and many women simply retreat from the ordeal and from themselves as feeling people. Other women are assailed by self-recrimination, self-disgust, guilt, horror, panic, fear of a recurrence, or a desire for violent retribution.

What to do if you are raped The immediate need of some women is to contact a close female friend or relative whom they totally trust and who can comfort them. For others it is more comfortable to talk over the experience with a stranger — a doctor or a policewoman. Despite your grief and shock, if you are a rape victim only you can know which of these choices is the right one for you; if at all possible, try to decide for yourself whether you want to seek medical or legal help, or both.

Your first natural impulse in such circumstances may well be to shower or bathe and put on fresh clothing in an attempt to assuage feelings of having been contaminated, or made unclean. But it is very important that you do neither of these things if you wish to press charges. (Of course, if clothing has been removed or badly torn you will nevertheless need to cover yourself.) Washing or changing could destroy important forensic evidence — for instance, an indication of the blood type of the rapist.

It is possible, however, to get help from a policewoman and see a doctor without necessarily making a formal complaint. Indeed, many women do prefer to avoid any legal follow-up because they feel that the procedure of pressing charges and going to court may be as distressing as the rape.

The legal situation is that a man must be regarded as innocent until proved guilty; any legal process is therefore bound to involve considerable stress and anguish for you as a rape victim. There will be questions designed to test your respectability and intentions, and you will be obliged to relive the incident in every detail. In Britain, this situation has improved a little since the institution of Rape Crisis Centres, but it is still a highly stressful ordeal. Crisis Centres are now available in most cities and are often open round the clock. Where they are not, there is usually a recorded message that includes the telephone number of a sympathetic doctor who can be contacted. Another useful option, run by several inner-city volunteer service organizations, is the Victims Support Scheme.

In addition, recent changes in legislation do afford rape victims some protection against excessive, insensitive or aggresive questioning and publicity. Remember: unless you do take legal proceedings against him, the rapist goes scot-free and will almost certainly rape again — and if he is personally known to you, it could be you he attacks for a second time. Whoever his victim happens to be, next time he may be even more violent.

The physical hazards of rape   It is sensible for every woman who has suffered rape to see a doctor as soon as possible after the attack. This is for the purpose of examination and treatment for any internal or external damage, tears or bruises, and for protection against possible later pregnancy or a sexually transmitted disease. If you are raped in mid-cycle there is a 30 per cent risk of becoming pregnant. Discuss this possibility with your doctor and ask for the morning-after pill, see page 31, which must be taken within 48 hours of the act of rape.

If you are raped by a stranger there is also the worrying possibility of having contracted a sexually transmitted disease, and this too should be discussed with your doctor. Treatment against this may include a high dose of penicillin or a 'cocktail' of doxycycline, ampicillin and metronidazole, followed at some later time by a blood test.

If you find the prospect of going for such an examination too daunting after your ordeal, take along a trusted friend or relative and insist that she be allowed to remain with you throughout the examination. In fact, it is advisable to have such support whether you feel you need it or not.

PREVENTING RAPE

Rape can happen to women of all ages: it does not happen only to nubile teenagers, or women in their 20s. It can happen to a little girl of three or four, or indeed, to a frail, elderly woman in her nineties; whatever age you are it could happen to you. So it makes sense to be on your guard against such a possibility and to take whatever steps you can to safeguard yourself.

That does not mean limiting your personal freedom to the point of not leaving your home after dark, or compulsively checking and re-checking every door and window morning, noon and night. But it does mean taking precautions instead.
For instance:
● Fit good locks on doors and windows, whether or not you live alone. Some rapists get their kicks from forcing your partner to watch, and he may be unprepared or no match for a night-time intruder, particularly an armed one.

Your local police station will be happy to send along a security expert to advise you on suitable locks.
● Establish good relations with your neighbours and, if you all have telephones, exchange numbers and keep these listed in a handy place; add to the list the number of your local police station and of your doctor.
● If you live alone, stay ex-directory or give only your initials for the phone directory so that it is not evident that you are female. If you have a name-tab by your doorbell, again give initials only.
● Fix a porch or door light, both back and front. Fit a spy-glass in both doors if there is easy access to the back of the house and never open up, even if expecting a caller, without first checking who is there.
● If the caller claims to be from, say, the Gas or Electricity Board or indeed, the police, keep the door on a chain until he has provided

proof of his authorization.
● If you are alone in the house *never* let strangers over the threshhold.
● If you are out alone and have the slightest suspicion that you are being followed, do not hesitate to walk up to the nearest house and ring the bell. No reasonable householder would object in such circumstances.
● Never take short cuts through ill-lit back streets or alleyways — better to be late than to be attacked and not arrive at all.
● Learn some form of self-defence if you possibly can — even a 'seven-stone weakling' can learn techniques for coping effectively with most assailants.

But, in extremis, remember that it is better to live through an ordeal than to resist and risk your life when the odds are clearly against you.

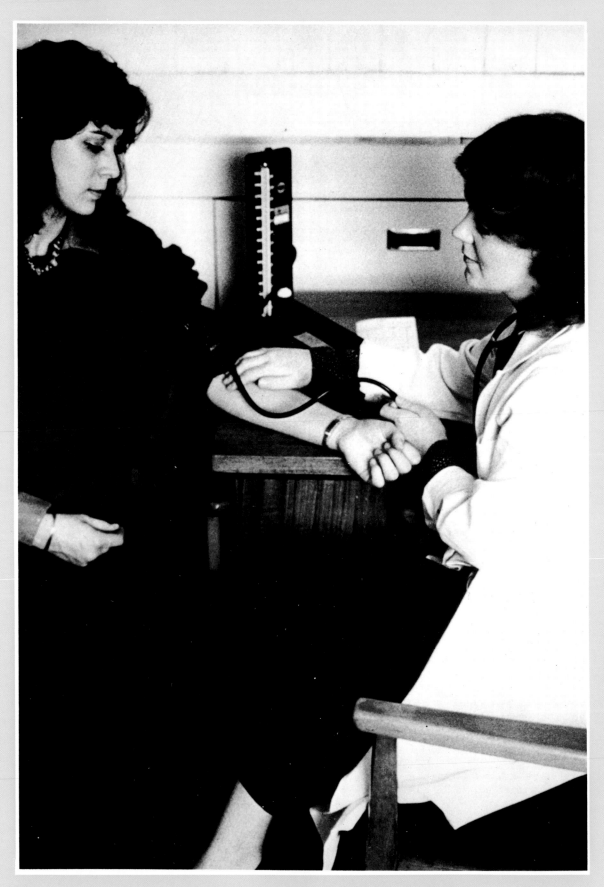

Health Care

● Choices in Health Care ● Your Medical Record ●
● Managing your Doctor ● Self-Help, Orthodox or Alternative Treatment ●
● Some Alternative Therapies ● Cancer

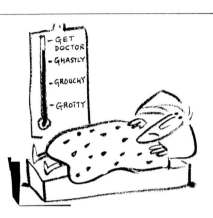

THE MEDICAL HISTORY of individual women can vary from needing to see a doctor just once or twice in 20 years or so, to twice-weekly visits to the surgery. Males and females on average have the same pattern of doctor attendance until they are about 12 years old, then women tend to visit their doctors far more often until their late forties, at which stage men start requiring treatment for the stress-related, degenerative diseases: heart disease, respiratory complaints, diabetes, digestive disorders, cancers. and so on.

The majority of women's consultations are concerned with birth control, childbirth and urogenital problems. Because of a woman's physical and biological make-up, she is likely to fall ill or need medical advice far more often than a man throughout her most active years. Even the healthiest woman is likely to find that she suffers from the occasional minor ailment, such as dysmenorrhea or thrush, varying in degrees from the irritating to the seriously debilitating. It is important, therefore, for every woman to be aware of this extra physical vulnerability and to know and understand her body fully, the way it functions, the risks she may run, the diseases she may catch and, finally, the different methods and techniques available in terms of treatment, so that she can make positive choices in her own health care. Self-knowledge can enable her to practice preventative medicine in the sense that by being aware of her life style choices she can do much to prevent serious diseases from 'ever developing.

Your health is your responsibility

This seems a self-evident truth but, in fact, it is a point that needs reiterating. In this age of medical experts and high technology we have lost a great deal of the basic knowledge previously passed down from one generation of women to the next, regarding daily health care and the home treatment of the simpler ailments. One of the aims of this chapter — and, indeed, this book — is to help you to care for yourself, treat basic disorders yourself and decide when and if you need general medical or specialist assistance.

There are times for us all when we feel we cannot cope any more, that we need help, either because we are ill, miserable, confused, or all three. At this point most women, if they do not have a close female friend or relative to advise and care for them, often turn instead to their doctor. However, a doctor is often not the right person to help. Hindered by overwork and by his very training, which does not encourage an understanding of people on a mutually equal basis, his ability is principally that of diagnosing recognized diseases and prescribing the appropriate medication.

A survey carried out in the late 1970s in London showed that more than 75 per cent of women every single day take some form of pill, either self-administered or prescribed by a doctor. And on a national basis, recent figures record that £21 million worth of mood-altering drugs, mostly tranquillizers, are prescribed yearly, three quarters of them for women. Why are so many women being given drugs to suppress and otherwise alter their moods and feelings — to make them sleep or to wake them up, to calm them down or cheer them up — when they go to their doctors with a wide range of complaints or disorders actually requiring more varied attention and care?

The present situation is this: women are taking their complaints to health care professionals who, by virtue of their very training, cannot understand them. For instance, if a woman complains to her doctor about pre-menstrual fluid retention, irrational rages or recurring breast pain, unless her symptoms fit in with a textbook description of a disease recognized by Western science the woman is often told that it is all in her mind and that she will either 'get over it' or 'it will pass' or to 'take some rest', or whatever. Alternatively, the doctor may prescribe a mood-altering drug. This last alternative is an attractive one for the busy doctor; he can send his patient away and both of them feel that something has been done, that the meeting was effective. Furthermore, the doctor is not likely to be bothered by the woman again, at least until the prescription runs out. It makes good sense, therefore, to know what other choices there are.

The choices in health care

Let us take the example of a woman with a vaginal discharge. There are many courses of action open to her — from exploring a whole range of alternative therapies to self care:

Self care	Professional health care
● Doing nothing and hoping it will go away. ● Douching with either tap water, mild vinegar solution or mild bicarbonate solution. ● Buying a pre-prepared cleansing douche from the chemist.	● Consulting her doctor. ● Attending a women's clinic, usually sited in a local community centre. ● Asking for advice at a family planning clinic. ● Going to the local hospital's department of sexually transmitted diseases (usually called Special Clinics). ● Choosing from the range of alternative therapies: homoeopathy, aromatherapy, nutritional advice, naturopathy, and so on.

These choices apply for all minor ailments. If a woman chooses professional health care, of whatever kind, she will need to reassess her decision to continue this treatment according to whether or not she has been satisfied by her first visit. This is very important. We all tend to be overawed by professionals, and this is particularly so for women. Many a woman has been told when she presents her own perception of what is wrong with her to the doctor: 'I am the doctor around here!' Some doctors tend to separate patients into 'good' patients — those who accept the diagnosis and treatment uncritically — and 'bad' patients — those who ask questions he or she cannot answer, or who present their own diagnosis. Many of us feel this instinctively when we visit them and behave accordingly, never daring to complain or argue. Many women therefore come away greatly dissatisfied with the meeting, but do not like to question the doctor's 'wisdom' or go elsewhere for

THE NEW GUIDE TO WOMEN'S HEALTH

Your medical record

FAMILY HISTORY

		Date
Mother (occupation)	Patricia Ann Housewife	b1928
Father (occupation)	Charles David Schoolteacher (died from stroke)	b1921 d1975
Sisters	Sarah Louise Schoolteacher (recurring migraine)	b1951
Brothers	David Arthur Representative (bronchitis)	b1953

IMMUNIZATION

	Date		Date
Diptheria	1954		
Polio	1954		
Typhoid	1954	1967	
Whooping cough			
German measles	1976		
Tuberculosis	1958		
Others			

PERSONAL HISTORY

	Date
Hospitalization/surgery	
Appendectomy	1966
Gall Bladder	1983
Chronic ailments	
Known allergies	
Hay fever .	
Recurring symptoms/common ailments	
Thrush / cystitis, Headaches .	
Long-term medication	

GYNAECOLOGICAL HISTORY

		Date
Age when periods started	13	1961
Are periods regular?	yes	
Sexual problems		
Miscarriages		
Abortions		
Sterilization		

METHODS OF CONTRACEPTION

		Date
Age when you started sex	18	1966
Methods of contraception		
Marvelon		1966
Brevinor		1972
Logynon		76/78 77/80

TESTS

	Date		Date
Blood pressure	120/70	Cervical smear	OK 1973
	1983		OK 1975
	120/70		OK 1976
	1984		OK 1978
			OK 1980
			OK 1981
			OK 1983
			OK 1984
ECG			OK 1985
Any other tests			
Eyes ok	1983		

CHILDREN

		Date
Pregnancies		78/79 81
Children (sex)		
Lisa Ann		2/7/77
David Thomas		5/9/81
Problems during birth		
Lisa - premature weight 4.11bs		

198

199

By keeping your own health record you will build up a personal medical history which will help jog your memory about such essential tests as cervical smears — all too easily forgotten.

The notes on your family history will show you which ailments may be hereditary — you should obviously be aware of these.

Remember that your personal health record is confidential — and should only be shown to those you trust.

help for fear of offending someone they see as a superior, or because they do not want to jeopardize what is essentially an important relationship, or to be dismissed as 'neurotic'.

Your medical record

Many of us have in our personal files documents that chart various stages in our physical and intellectual development, but often there is no record of immunization, childhood ailments or hospital admissions. At a major London teaching hospital, patients are encouraged to keep their own maternity records. This enables fathers-to-be and other members of the family to follow the progress of the pregnancy with the expectant mother. It also follows that the pregnant woman will be better motivated towards taking iron tablets and following a sensible diet if she feels that she is responsible for her health.

When you have some spare time, sit down and fill out as much of your medical record as you can, starting at birth. Take stock of the contents and advice in this book and decide if there are any common tests that you need. A basic check-up by a doctor should cover such things as breast examination, blood pressure, cervical smear and testing the heart and other major organs. Most family planning clinics and health centres are very helpful with check-ups and they are keen to promote preventative medicine. Once you have established a personal health record, you can log results of tests and X-rays and details of vaccinations. It goes without saying that a personal health record is confidential and should only be shown to those people in whom you have complete trust.

How to manage your doctor

Women have been brought up to be 'good girls': if they are good they will be given the sweetie, do well, be loved, attract a husband or, in this case, get better. The doctor is the Western equivalent of the primitive wise-man-cum-witch-doctor, and to offend him will, women instinctively feel, bring his wrath down upon them. That is, to go against the doctor's prescriptions will automatically result in their illness getting worse, or, at the very least, not clearing up or getting better.

None of this is intended to suggest that doctors are consciously power-seekers, or malicious, or uncaring or even unsympathetic. The relationship is one of collusion: the patient wants the doctor to be all-powerful and all-knowing just as much as the doctor may need to assume this role. And just as many women are today challenging this state of affairs, so many doctors, too,

What your prescription means *Under the terms of the National Health Service, your doctor prescribes a drug by writing a prescription which you take to a chemist or pharmacist. If your doctor specifies the 'generic' name, he or she will put BP or BPC after it. Each drug has only one generic name but may have several trade names — this is because it may be manufactured by many different companies.*

If the patient is under 12 his or her age must be entered here.

The name and address of the patient is entered by the doctor.

NP stands for 'nomen proprium', Latin for 'proper name'. This tells the pharmacist to put either the generic or brand name on the container. If NP is crossed out the pharmacist leaves out the name of the drug.

A traditional symbol for the word 'recipe'.

This number tells the pharmacist how many tablets to put in the container.

The official stamp gives the name and address of the doctor plus the name of the local Family Practitioners Committee.

The length of time for which the drug should be taken.

The pharmacist writes in this column the name and quantity of the drug dispensed.

The Pricing Bureau — who refund the pharmacist with the cost of the prescription — make notes in this column.

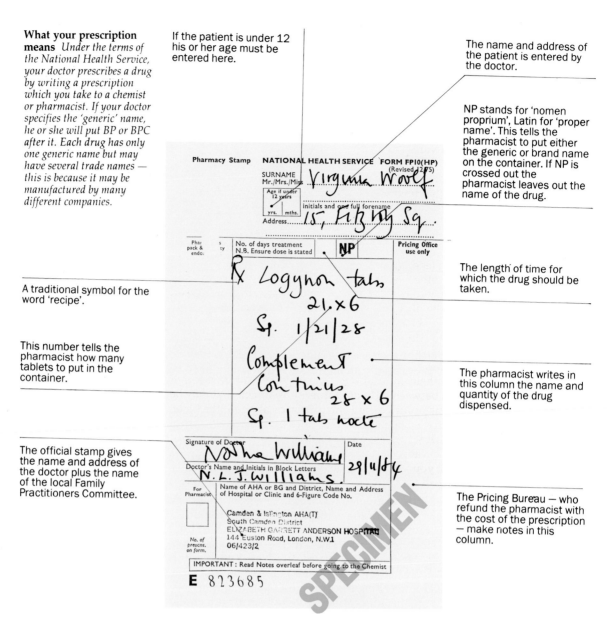

are weary of being set on the pedestal, always having to know the answers. It must also be said, that when the relationship works, and both patient and doctor cooperate towards a happy conclusion, it can be very satisfying to both of them. Both feel that they have fulfilled their roles well: the patient feels cared for by someone who knows more than she does and the doctor feels the satisfaction of having cared and cured.

Your first visit

In every human interaction each of us brings, as it were, a portfolio of gifts and a portfolio of needs to the meeting. Both portfolios of each person must be recognized. So, just as the doctor needs to recognize what his patient has to offer in the way of knowledge and insight (because each woman is the expert on her own body), so the patient must be aware of the doctor's need to practise the skills he or she possesses, and to be verbally supported in his or her effectiveness. Doctors must learn to listen and patients must learn to give appropriate information on their condition so that they may have an informed say in whatever treatment is prescribed and undergone.

This is the most important factor in a good patient/doctor relationship and lays the foundation for future consultations no matter how serious or life-threatening the disease processes are.

As the patient, your first meeting with your doctor or other health care professional you choose to visit with your problem will be much more satisfying if you state exactly what is troubling you, clearly and directly. Think about this beforehand and make a note of any points, dates and symptoms that are (or may be) relevant. If, for example, you have abdominal pain, it is useful to be able to state quite clearly:

- When you first became aware of it.
- Exactly where it is.
- The things that make it better and the things that make it worse.

The doctor may then ask if you have ever had a similar condition before and, if so, what sort of treatment was helpful then. If it is a recurrence and treatment was by the same doctor, he may simply refer to your medical record — but be prepared for such questions if you can, and have dates and details of treatment ready.

If this line of questioning leads the doctor to a working diagnosis, he will then ask you about certain other elements in your life, such as appetite and sleep, and examine you to try to rule out the possible serious causes of pain. He will then tell you what the likely diagnosis is, and which specific form of treatment he feels will be of help to you. Alternatively, if his examination finds a condition that needs further investigation he will ask you to undergo X-rays or blood tests, as appropriate. At this point it is essential for you to understand clearly what these tests are for. Ask your doctor for a clear description of the tests and their implications. You need this information to help you make any decision between different forms of treatment that may be suggested to you, so *do* persist until you are completely clear about the issue.

If, after your meeting with the doctor, you have other questions or worries, either go back a second time or write your doctor a brief letter setting them out clearly; enclose a stamped, self-addressed envelope and ask him to provide the information you require. If you do not receive a reply within a reasonable time, phone the surgery or call there. Do not be discouraged or give up. It is your health that is involved and it is in your best interests to persist.

After your first visit, you will either come away from the meeting satisfied and decide to follow the treatment prescribed until your problem clears up, or you will come away feeling dissatisfied with the meeting and/or the treatment suggested. If further communication by letter or telephone does not help, then you must decide how and where you wish to seek a second opinion.

Most doctors intuitively realize when they have failed to communicate adequately with a patient and at this point are often happy to suggest to the patient that she receive a second opinion. In general practice a doctor may suggest that one of his partners see the patient or that she have an extended interview with a health visitor or the practice nurse. Alternatively, if it is a single-handed practice, the patient may be referred to the local hospital, or she may visit another doctor and ask to be transferred.

Recent legislation has set up a number of bodies in the health care field which patients have recourse to if they are unhappy with their treatment — among them the Patients Association (see page 203). If you are *not* treated with respect and compassion by your physician, you are entitled to make a change. It is wise to do this in a calm, sensible atmosphere, and is often best done by letter. Your relationship with your doctor is not binding, you can opt out of it at any time, and if you are unhappy with your doctor it is better to seek out another practitioner rather than live with your doubts and dissatisfaction. A local post office normally has a list of all doctors in practice in its area, but this is a rather hit-or-miss method of selecting alternative help in that the list obviously gives no guidance on what individual doctors are like. Ask women friends and acquaintances for their recommendations, just as you might when seeking professional help of any kind. If, on a visit to your prospective new doctor, he or she agrees to accept you as a patient, any necessary transfer of documents such as medical records can be arranged by post, without the need for a further visit to your former doctor.

A further option is to seek alternative health care. This may be in the form of any one of a number of therapies outlined in the following pages or, with routine disorders, self-treatment.

Self-help, orthodox or alternative treatment?

Increasingly over the last few decades, medical knowledge and responsibility for health care has become concentrated on specialists and general practitioners. People have got into the habit of turning to their doctor the moment anything ails them. This is now changing in Britain because of the sheer overburdening of the resources of the National Health Service, which has brought about an increasing interest in preventative medicine and in self-help. Also, disenchantment with the wonders of modern science and drug technology has made great numbers of people turn to alternative forms of treatment, exploring not only the more well-known therapies such as homoeopathy, osteopathy and acupuncture but also more unusual forms such as aromatherapy.

Although this diversification and loosening of our reliance on the overworked and necessarily limited doctor is an entirely good thing, the present enthusiasm for alternative therapies may create a situation of complete polarization between conventional and alternative medicine. What is needed is a holistic approach: that is, the notion that no therapy is either right or wrong in itself, but all therapies, from antibiotics to herbs, should have a place in the treatment of the whole person, because what is appropriate for one person in one situation may be inappropriate in another. At the moment, for instance, medical thinking puts considerable emphasis on dietary change — particularly cutting the intake of fats — as vital in the prevention of coronary heart disease. Whereas it is no bad thing for all of us to lower our fats consumption — which at present runs at an average of 42 per cent of our calorie intake — it is important to remember that the majority of studies on the incidence of heart disease and the effect of diet in its control have been conducted on men. We ought therefore to be wary of blanket pronouncements on what women should or should not eat because men and women have very different nutritional requirements. It may thus be entirely appropriate for *men* to radically cut their fat intake, yet it is a fact that, due to the large amounts of oestrogen women have to metabolize, their need for dietary fat is greater than the amount men need.

Many people today do not realize that medical advice and treatment is not dispensed solely by doctors and hospitals. Many different sources of treatment and advice are available — pharmacists, nurses, social workers, as well as self-help and support groups for specific problems and diseases.

It is important that women should be aware of all the different possibilities in health care and, instead of getting locked into a frustrating battle with the system, take advantage of the wide variety of resources available. It is time and cost effective, liberating and self-empowering to turn to the right person for advice and treatment at the right time. It is satisfying to receive the help you really need rather than to go away miserable and dissatisfied from your doctor or health care practitioner because he or she has not been able to help you and has been obliged to come up with a cover-all solution.

Nevertheless, the choice in medical care today is certainly bewildering. When should you opt for acupuncture rather than for pills? When is it appropriate to have surgery rather than homoeopathic treatment? When is your doctor the best source of help and when is it better to seek help from a pharmacist, psychotherapist or nutritional adviser? All these and many more questions are now being asked. There are no easy answers, because it all comes down to what is appropriate for each individual in each separate case and at different times in the same individual's life. However, the following guidelines can help you to make up your mind which is the right therapy or care for your situation.

Below is a brief description of some of the alternative therapies that have become widely established and are fairly easily accessible. If you feel you could be helped by one of these, it is wise to find out more about the particular therapy before seeking out a therapist; this will better enable you to assess the experience and skill of the therapist and whether this particular therapy really is suitable for you. It is always advisable to seek a qualified practitioner of whatever therapy you choose.

There are many good books available on the different therapies as well as organizations that can advise you.

Some alternative therapies

In autumn 1983, the British Holistic Medical Association was set up to bridge the gap between orthodox medical bodies and the growing number of practitioners of alternative therapies. Many present at the inaugural conference felt unhappy with the classing of therapies such as acupuncture as 'alternative' and preferred the adjective 'complementary'. After all, the crux of holistic medicine is that different therapies work together to provide appropriate individual health care; orthodox medicine and other therapies are by no means mutually exclusive.

There are, however, just as many practitioners of 'alternative therapy' who feel that their system of health care provides a genuine alternative to the orthodox medical system based on drugs and surgical technology, and do not feel that they can work comfortably in conjunction with Western medicine.

Some naturopaths, for instance, require their patients to forgo all drugs and to follow strict dietary regimes and other natural treatments. They feel that their treatments cannot work if the body is still having to cope with foreign substances such as chemical drugs. Detoxification to allow the body's own natural healing systems to come fully into play is a basic principle of naturopathy. Similarly, some homoeopaths feel that their treatment cannot be effective in conjunction with antibiotics and other synthetic drugs in that their remedies work subtly with the body's own immune system and would be obliterated by powerful doses of Western medicine.

The discussion as to whether other therapies should be called 'alternative' or 'complementary' will doubtless continue, but if we are to take the principle of holism literally we, as the patients, should consider both orthodox *and* alternative therapies as having validity for us.

As we become familiar with different 'alternative' therapies we may find that we prefer to use one, or two, forms of therapy more and more exclusively, and decide that they work better for us in terms of general health care and treatment of minor ailments than conventional drugs. Surgery, too, has a place in holism. Breast surgery and Caesarian sections have saved many women's lives. Not everything that is 'natural' is automatically good and not everything produced by modern society is bad. However, the principal difference between modern medicine and the 'alternative' therapies is that the first treats disease and the second treats people. It is people who get ill, not individual parts of the person (for instance, their stomach or their cells).

It is because orthodox medicine tends to treat the symptoms of an illness rather than the deeper cause that it has only a limited success in many diseases and ailments prevalent in our society: mental disorders, cancers, heart disease, muscular and neurological disorders, digestive malfunctions and so on. Holistic therapies start with the person, the individual, who has the disorder rather than with specific symptoms. They take into account the patient's temperament, life history — including early illnesses and illnesses of their parents — past and present relationships, lifestyle, work and recreational activities, attitudes, and emotional and psychological

Holism

indications. By building up a detailed picture of the patient as an individual, they can base their treatment on what they feel will work for that particular person rather than on what is indicated as effective against a particular virus or bacteria.

Another principle of holistic systems of medicine is that we all have the will and the capacity to heal ourselves if our immune system is encouraged and properly strengthened. Many therapies — such as acupuncture and homoeopathy — thus work largely by 'tuning up', as it were, the body's own defences and antibodies. Conventional drug therapy treats the patient as a passive recipient of medication that supplants the body's own immune system and attacks the virus or bacteria causing the illness. Of course, drugs are themselves invasive and perceived by the immune system as foreign substances which are toxic and so have to be coped with. This often creates double the work for the body, which is also trying to fend off the virus causing the illness. Many drugs render the immune system inoperative or greatly weakened, which is why people often get colds, flu or stomach or vaginal disorders following a course of antibiotics.

Homoeopathy

A holistic system of medicine founded by Dr Samuel Hahnemann in the early 1800s, homoeopathy works on the principles of like-curing-like and that remedies given in very great dilution may be more effective than a full strength medicine. (Both these principles are similar to those of

Homoeopathy was founded early in the nineteenth-century by Dr Samuel Hahnemann, a German physician who became disillusioned with the medical practises of the day. His desk, chair, books and cases of remedies are preserved at the Royal Homoeopathic Hospital in London, where it is possible to receive homoeopathic treatment under the health service.

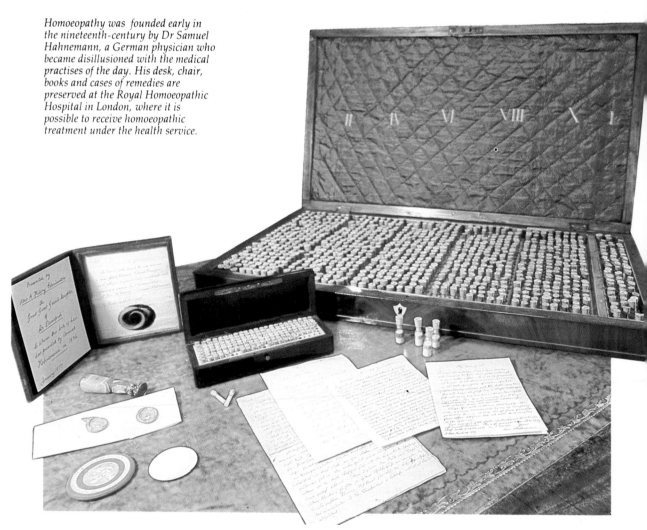

46

immunization.) The medication is gradually diluted to less than one part in a million through a process of intense shaking called 'succussion' until barely a molecule of the original drug is left. This has caused homoeopathy to be much ridiculed by the orthodox medical profession, although it is now well established, with many practitioners and several hospitals in the UK. Treatment is available on the National Health Service.

The underlying concept of homoeopathy is that we all have a 'vital force' within us and are capable of healing ourselves (except in the case of disorders requiring surgery) if given a nudge in the right direction. Indeed, the symptoms are seen as part of the body's attempt to shrug off the disease. Current research remains inconclusive, largely because there are so many factors involved in recovering from an illness that it is difficult to isolate the effects of any one drug or remedy and ascertain its exact role in that recovery. However, homoeopathy has helped many people. All the remedies used are naturally occurring, mostly as plants and tend to have fewer side effects than modern conventional drugs.

A homoeopath acts very similarly to a doctor dealing with the same ailments and maladies. However, homoeopathy does not claim to be exclusive and homoeopaths will recommend other approaches and therapies if they feel this is necessary. The first consultation is always lengthy because the doctor must build up a picture of you as a person, your general physical and emotional state and any environmental pressures you may be under, on the principle that all illnesses have a psychosomatic element. In this it successfully bridges the gap between physical and psychiatric medicine. Homoeopathy is also suitable for disorders that affect more than one body system and is successful in dealing with addictions, such as alcoholism, and for those with allergies or hypersensitivity to drugs.

Just as in the case of some immunizations, treatment can initially cause the patient to feel an intensification of the symptoms usually associated with the particular illness — but this passes as the treatment begins to work positively.

Naturopathy

By definition, naturopathy is treatment that uses nothing that does not come from within the patient. Naturopaths use a number of different methods to help the individual — principally fasting, prescriptive diets, hydrotherapy, general restorative and body-building methods and psychotherapy. Each patient is treated as an individual with different needs rather than a collection of disorders. Nature cure has a long and well-established tradition but has recently seen a popular revival as eminent doctors in specialist medicine — such as the treatment of cancer — have started to achieve successes with dietary and fasting measures where orthodox drugs have failed. The methods fall outside the knowledge of most doctors, although some are now extending their training into these areas.

Naturopathy is based on three main principles:
- That all forms of disease are due to the same cause: the accumulation in the body through years of wrong living (faulty breathing, eating and drinking) of waste materials and toxins. Fasting and cleansing diets aim to rid the body of this refuse so that the healing process can begin.
- That the body has an in-built recognition of, and is always striving for, health. Symptoms of disease, such as colds and coughs, are the body's attempt to throw off the accumulated wastes and the invading bacteria. Orthodox drugs, by treating only the symptoms merely suppress them, to reappear another time.
- That the body contains the ability to heal itself and return to health provided it is given the right help.

The last two principles are similar to those of homoeopathy. Whereas homoeopathy has a well-established system of medication, however, naturopaths differ widely in the fasts, diets and treatments they favour. There is also a wide range of naturopathic institutions (health farms) to choose from, and it is wise before going to a therapist to seek advice or recommendation from someone you trust.

Naturopathy has been particularly successful in the treatment of such conditions as digestive and liver problems, haemorrhoids, colitis, gastritis, sore throats and bronchial conditions. It has also been used for more serious illnesses. Some naturopathic doctors are expert diagnosticians and can refer patients to surgeons and oncologists (cancer experts) if they feel that their skills are insufficient to deal with the individual patients' needs.

Acupuncture

Acupuncture is one of the most ancient forms of medicine, and originated in China. The word 'acupuncture' means 'needle puncture', a discipline that is practised today in China alongside Western medicine. About one in five surgical procedures there are carried out using acupuncture as a substitute for chemical anaesthesia.

The technique involves inserting fine needles to just below the skin at specific points on any of the 12 main 'meridians' (energy pathways) that run through the body. These control the lung, large bowel, stomach, spleen, heart, small bowel, bladder, kidney, the membrane that encloses the heart, 'triple warmer', gall-bladder and liver. Down the centre front and centre back of the body are two further meridians, making 14 in all.

Because these meridians do not correspond to the nervous system, acupuncture has drawn a great deal of derision in the past from Western doctors who failed to see how the technique could possibly be effective. Yet, despite the lack of conclusive clinical trials, acupuncture has become more and more accepted in the West by virtue of its evident success in relieving pain and symptoms. It is used more and more to relieve headaches, migraines, neck and back problems and other muscle and joint pains. It has also been found helpful in neurological disorders, menstrual pain, and with conditions such as sinusitis, hay fever, asthma, and stomach, bowel and bladder disorders. It has helped those who wish to stop smoking and lose weight, and particularly in general 're-conditioning' of the body, when convalescing after a debilitating, possibly long-term, illness.

A first consultation with an acupuncturist is always quite lengthy because the therapist needs information on your lifestyle, eating habits, sensitivity to cold and heat, and so on. The acupuncturist may feel that your problem is not suitable for this therapy, but if it is, treatment will be decided according to your needs as an individual and may, for example, comprise twice-weekly sessions of 45 minutes.

Some people find the insertion of the needles painless, others feel a twinge, and others report a sharp, momentary pain. Several needles are likely to be used at different points on the body and left in place for a few minutes or even up to half an hour. The points of insertion are not necessarily anywhere near the problem area: a headache sufferer, for instance, may have needles inserted in her feet. Sometimes symptoms temporarily worsen after treatment, but this usually clears within hours, or at most days.

Exactly how acupuncture works has yet to be determined; several interesting and plausible theories have been tested and ruled out. But research in the United States has shown that acupuncture does cause the brain to produce endorphins (pain-relieving substances), and what is certain is that acupuncture *does* work. Some medical practitioners in this country now practise acupuncture and there is a Medical Acupuncture Society.

Chiropractic and osteopathy

Both chiropractic and osteopathy are manipulative therapies that focus on mechanical disorders of the joints, particularly the spine. The theory behind both practices is that many of the disorders patients suffer stem from abnormalities and strains in the body's structure rather than from trauma, degeneration or inflammation. Abnormal function may be due to early damage, undue stress either physical (as in sports) or mental, or bad posture

TECHNIQUES OF ACUPUNCTURE

Acupuncture involves puncturing the skin with round-tipped needles that push aside blood vessels so they are not pierced. Sometimes, the needles may be inserted to a depth of an inch or so, either at tender points or at apparently unrelated ones (see main text), and left in for up to 20 minutes, with some manipulation. Up to 15 points may be stimulated at a session.

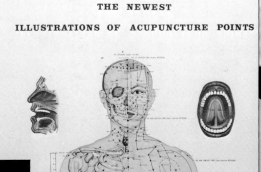

THE NEWEST
ILLUSTRATIONS OF ACUPUNCTURE POINTS

①

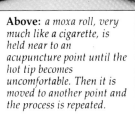

Above: although acupuncture points are usually stimulated with needles of stainless steel, other methods are practised. Moxibustion involves stimulating points with moxa (Artemisia japonica or dried mugwort). Here a moxa 'cork' sends heat along the needle into a point.

Above: a moxa roll, very much like a cigarette, is held near to an acupuncture point until the hot tip becomes uncomfortable. Then it is moved to another point and the process is repeated.

Below: in acupressure, or cupping, a vacuum is made by burning off air inside a beaker with a swab of methylated spirits and the inverted cup is then placed over a point, drawing the covered skin into the cup.

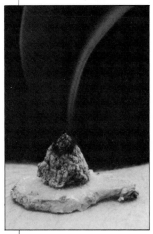

Left: small, slow burning cones of moxa are positioned over the acupuncture points so that they are warmed gently.

COMMON DISORDERS: INTEGRATING THERAPIES

Listed below are some integrating therapies for a number of common complaints.

MENSTRUAL DISORDERS

Self-help Vitamin Therapy: Vitamin B_6 and Vitamin E.

Acupuncture Works through neurological channels to alleviate pain.

Aromatherapy and colour therapy Work through the two powerful senses of smell and sight to counteract symptoms.

Biofeedback Cultivates awareness of autonomic nervous system, and teaches relaxation techniques.

Herbalism Extracts of sage or oil of evening primrose, camomile tea.

Homoeopathy Valerian or other remedies, after evaluation of general health of patient.

Naturopathy Detoxification following dietary advice.

Orthodox Anti-prostaglandin drugs such as aspirin and non-steroidal anti-inflammatory agents.

Surgery Dilatation and curettage (D&C).
It is always better to try alternative and drug therapies before resorting to this last extreme, for a D&C leaves scars in the cervix which could cause problems in pregnancy.

Yoga and Meditation Encourages relaxation of muscle spasm and inner awareness.

MIGRAINE

Self-help Breathing exercises; avoidance of trigger foods, such as chocolate and cheese.

Biofeedback and meditation To calm and re-train the nervous system.

Herbalism Treatment with the feverfew plant has proved particularly successful.

Homoeopathy Herbal medicines prescribed after evaluation of individual.

Naturopathy Vegetarianism and a variety of detoxification methods and herbal remedies.

Orthodox Beta-blockers — modern drugs that slow nerve tissue response.

DEPRESSION AND ANXIETY

Self-help Exercise to increase oxygen intake and encourage the body's own release of endorphins (natural pain relievers).

Assertiveness training Develops sense of self and own strengths.

Counselling A variety of different resources exist from the relatively informal one of confiding problems to a friend, to organized psychotherapeutic interviews.

Naturopathy Detoxification and discovery of any allergens, trigger foods or addictions.

Orthodox Anti-depressant drugs, electro-convulsion therapy (a highly controversial treatment usually reserved for very serious, recurring depression, but it can be very effective).

Vitamin therapy High doses of vitamins B and C.

Yoga and relaxation To encourage inner peace and sense of calmness.

UROLOGICAL PROBLEMS

Self-help Greatly increase fluid intake; gently douche and urinate after sex; neutralize acid/alkaline balance by eating and drinking alkaline foods and drinks such as barley water.

Herbalism Uva Ursi tablets, herbal tisanes.

Naturopathy and homoeopathy Dietary and holistic psycho-social investigation and advice.

Orthodox Wide variety of antibiotics.

VAGINITIS

Self-help Two fingerfuls of live active yoghurt inserted into vagina for three days at end of period; gently douche after sex; stop using bubble baths or washing underwear with biological detergents; wear cotton underwear rather than synthetic so that greater circulation of air is allowed in vaginal area.

Homoeopathy A variety of herbal medicines prescribed as appropriate for the individual.

Naturopathy Vegetarian and other alkalinizing diets.

Orthodox A variety of antibiotics and anti-fungal treatments, taken orally or as pessaries.

or locomotion. The symptoms must be treated before they develop into actual damage to body structure.

There is also mounting evidence that problems of the internal organs may be related to distortions of the spine and other joints. (Certainly Alexander teachers (see page 106), have always believed this, but maintain that the body must be re-trained rather than simply having the symptoms removed through manipulation, since they will only return if the individual continues the postural habits which led to the problem in the first place.)

The main differences between the two therapies is that chiropractic (now one of the most widely recognized 'alternative' treatments) makes use of X-rays as part of the diagnostic procedure whereas osteopathy relies on observation, touch and a lengthy consultation, which aims to assess all elements of the patient's lifestyle that may contribute to his or her problem. Roughly speaking, today chiropractors are more numerous than osteopaths. Osteopathy is now widely accepted as a useful and effective therapy to which many doctors refer patients. It is suitable for musculo-skeletal complaints, backache, neck pain, headaches (many problems originating from the spine may produce their 'ache' in other muscles, for example in the leg or arm), and for a variety of problems relating to posture. As such it is of special relevance to women since they are particularly prone to such disorders. Over one third of all women in the UK will consult a doctor at some time in their lives for the very common problem of back pain.

One word of caution: anyone contemplating treatment by either chiropractic or osteopathy should seek out a qualified person — there are dangers in either discipline if put into practice by an unskilled practitioner.

Biofeedback and autogenic training

Both of these therapies teach the patient to exercise mind over matter. Similar in principle to the relaxation and meditation techniques described on page 103, biofeedback and autogenic training (AT) are also very effective stress management techniques.

Biofeedback uses electronic instruments to make the patient aware of his or her internal responses. The patient is connected by surface electrodes to a machine designed to feed back information on such body functions as heart rate, blood pressure, skin temperature, brain wave pattern or muscle tension. With the help of this information and a therapist, the patient learns to control these functions through trial and error. For example, some migraine sufferers have noted that their hands get cold before an attack. By learning to increase the temperature of their hands, perhaps simply by imagining a hot sun and thinking that their hands are getting warmer, they can avert an attack.

Autogenic training also utilizes the power of the mind to alter body responses. Essentially, it is a training in relaxation technique which switches off the arousal mechanism, or stress response implicated in stress-related disorders such as insomnia, tension, headaches, circulatory disorders, or heart and blood pressure problems.

Both therapies must be taught by trained practitioners and are not easily available on the NHS.

Other therapies

There are many other alternative therapies that you may wish to explore, such as herbalism, aromatherapy, reflexology, radionics, bioenergetics, and so on. It is always wise to read about them first and there are plenty of good books on these subjects. But there are not always regulatory and advisory bodies for all the therapies, so in such instances follow the advice of someone you trust or write for information and advice to either the British Holistic Medical Association or the College of Health in London. (The College of Health issues a periodical called *Self Health* and will be happy to advise you on any aspect of self help, alternative and orthodox medicine.)

Cancer

Cancer is a condition caused by malformed cells which have grown into solid lumps or tumours, which cause the destruction of normal tissue, result in pain and haemorrhage and also interrupt the normal functions of the tissues. Many scientists believe that cancer clones occur all over the body but are mopped up by good defence mechanisms before they actually cause disease. There is increasing interest not only in the lethal effects of smoking, but also in other environmental hazards such as asbestos and contamination of foodstuffs by insecticides used to spray crops. However, because of good sanitary hygiene and clean water we are not at risk to certain diseases like hepatitis which cause liver cancer and early death in many developing countries.

Cancer of the breast — with lung cancer fast catching up — is one of the

THE LANGUAGE OF CANCER

The following terms and expressions are used in connection with cancer and breast cancer in particular.

Biopsy: the removal of a small amount of tissue for laboratory examination.

Frozen section: a sample of the tissue removed for biopsy is frozen and placed under a microscope while you are under anaesthetic. If malignant cells are detected, the cancerous tissue is then removed. It is not always accurate so never consent to having an immediate mastectomy if the frozen section appears to show malignancy.

Fine needle aspiration: a needle is inserted into the breast to withdraw fluid for examination; a **needle biopsy** is a similar procedure. This procedure takes place without an anaesthetic.

Lumpectomy: an open biopsy in which·a semi-curved incision — usually between one and three inches — is made following the contours of the breast (so that it will heal well), and the suspect lump is removed for examination. This procedure may be combined with removal of lymph nodes from the armpit.

Mastectomy: the surgical removal of a breast. If the cancer is found in good time a very small amount of the breast may be removed rather than the whole breast.

Modified mastectomy: the affected breast tissue is removed plus some of the tissues in the armpit; a check is then made of how many lymph nodes (glands under the arm) are affected.

Sub-total mastectomy: in this operation approximately half of the breast is removed.

Other treatments
In some areas mastectomy is the only known technique for dealing with breast cancer, but an increasing number of patients (80 per cent in New York and 20 per cent in London) are now being offered other treatments. If you wish to pursue a different line of treatment you should visit an **oncologist**, a doctor who specializes in cancer.

He or she will be able to discuss with you the advantages and disadvantages of the following which may be used in combination with surgery or on their own — depending on the case:

Radiotherapy: radioactive rays are directed at the affected area. Side-effects can include burning of the skin and scarring; some women object to the permanent purple dye used to mark the 'fields' (target areas) of the radiation. There may also be nausea, fatigue, lethargy and depression.

Chemotherapy: treatment with very powerful drugs which can produce similar side-effects to radiotherapy. In addition there may also be hair loss or baldness.

Hormone therapy: this may be offered in addition to radiation and chemotherapy; depending on the individual it may be used on its own. Side-effects (apart from nausea) are fewer; some women have no side-effects at all.

The way forward?
The current work on personality and cancer survival does indicate that calm and resolute patients who understand their illness have a longer life expectancy than those who try to deny it or feel sorry for themselves. The keynote sentiment for both patients and doctors is one of cautious optimism with open, friendly discussions about each stage of diagnosis and treatment.

major causes of death in women. The figures, however, do show a slight improvement in the last couple of years, with 12,672 deaths from breast cancer recorded in the United Kingdom in 1983 compared to 13,980 deaths in 1981. With early detection and treatment the chances of recovering from the disease are good.

Breast cancer

The breast health examination The most important reason for examining your own body regularly is that by doing so you become thoroughly familiar with what is normal for you. Women's breasts — and women's bodies too — come in all shapes, sizes and textures, but once you are familiar with your own 'normal' body, you will quickly notice if any irregularity occurs and can seek medical advice.

The best way to learn how to examine your own breasts for any suspicious lumps is to be shown by someone who has been expertly taught. Every doctor who is interested in prevention can instruct you on how to examine your own breasts, but if you prefer not to go to your doctor, do visit a women's clinic or one of the early diagnostic centres.

When to examine your breasts The best time to examine your breasts is when you are in a shower, a bath or a warm bed, when you are most likely to be completely relaxed. Many of the instruction leaflets also suggest that you carry out this examination after your period because some of the tenderness and swelling which usually occurs towards the end of the cycle due to fluid retention will then not obscure any other bodily changes. However, one of the drawbacks of teaching women to do it after their period every month is that when they stop having periods — either because they are past the menopause, have had a hysterectomy or are in a period of stress — they forget to continue to examine their breasts. It is vital to examine your breasts monthly, regardless of age, and it is a good idea to do it at different times in your cycle.

One very good way of organizing this is to examine yourself on the first of every month, so that you know exactly when you last examined your breasts, and it will become a regular habit. It will also mean that you carry out this health check at many different times during your menstrual cycle, whether this is every 25, 28, 30 days or whatever.

Causes and risk factors During this century there has been much debate about, and research into, what can be the causes of breast cancer. Even in the nineteenth century it was known that women who had never had children were rather more likely to have breast cancer than those who had had a family. But there are other factors that appear to increase the risk:
● It definitely increases with age.
● If your mother or other female blood relative has, or had, cancer the likelihood is increased.
● If you have, or have had, any other form of cancer yourself, whether of the breast, the womb or an ovary, then that too is sometimes said to make your chances of developing breast cancer somewhat higher.
● If several members of your family have had different forms of cancer, then it is wise to be diligent about all the things that you can do to protect yourself — and breast self-examination is certainly one of them.
● Women who have had many chest X-rays as a child, or have had radiation therapy on the chest wall (although not many women have this now) are at increased risk.
● If you have had multiple biopsies so that you have a lot of scar tissue in the

WHERE AND HOW TO EXAMINE YOUR BREASTS

Start by placing the hand opposite to the breast you are examining high up in the armpit of one breast, where you will find a hollow space. Then, slowly bring your fingers down, gently but firmly along the edges of the breast tissue. Breasts often feel quite stringy in what is called the axillary tail, but if you do this every month you will recognize what is normal for you.

Next, use the flat of your hand to push each part of the breast against the rib cage.

Repeat the action with your fingertips and you will be able to detect any alterations in the actual texture or shape of the tissues. Most women's breasts are symmetrical, but with one slightly larger than the other. To make lumps easier to feel, stretch the breast tissue by extending the arm you are not using behind your head.

About 40 per cent of women have chronic lumpy breasts — that is, cystic swellings or bumpy areas

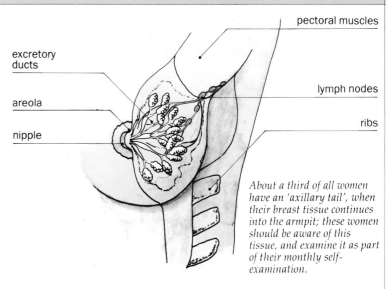

About a third of all women have an 'axillary tail', when their breast tissue continues into the armpit; these women should be aware of this tissue, and examine it as part of their monthly self-examination.

called fibro-adenosis. These women need to know which bumps are 'normal' (and therefore harmless) for them, and which they should keep a watchful eye on. This can only be done by self-check-ups.

Another good way to examine your breasts is to look in the mirror while you put on your bra. As you bend slightly forward to put it on, look in the mirror and observe

whether the nipples are reasonably symmetrical or whether there is any dimpling or change. Then, having fastened your bra, place your hand inside the cup so that you can gently lift up your breast, so that it fits neatly into the bra cup. In so doing, again you can feel for any irregularity. Incidentally, your bra should always be a perfect fit, without wiring or shaping.

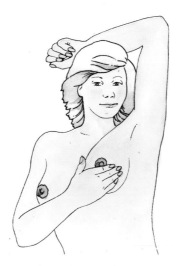

Place your finger tips in the hollow of your opposite armpit. The space there is clean and empty. Gradually bring your fingers down over the muscles.

Move your finger tips in a circular pattern, checking the whole breast. If you find a small, hard lump — like an uncooked grain of rice — then consult your doctor.

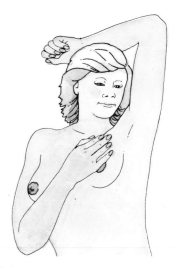

Place the flat of your hand over all the segments of your breasts in turn, crushing the breast tissue against the rib cage.

In the last five years, x-ray machines, or mammograms, have been specially designed to give the minimal radiation dosage by using accurate focusing beams and equipment that can be adjusted to fit each individual woman. The x-ray picture enables the radiologist to diagnose both benign and malignant changes in breast tissue.

The mammogram prevents unnecessary biopsies, and can detect changes that may be characteristic of early cancer before a lump has appeared or the patient herself is aware of it. Like self-examination, the mammogram is a further screening technique.

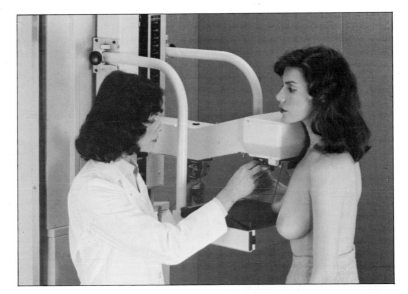

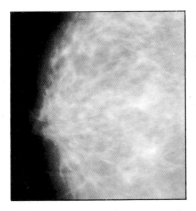

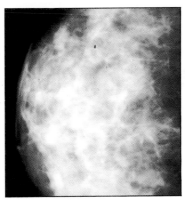

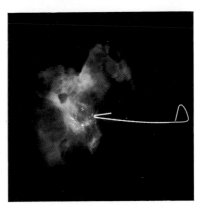

The first mammogram shows a normal breast. The heavy lines, representing the ducts, are symmetrical and regular.

This mammogram shows an abnormal area with disturbed ducts and micro-calcification which could be indicative of an early cancer. (To fight cancer cells the body naturally produces calcium.)

The suspicious area has been identified with a silver wire; injection of a blue dye will make the lesion even more obvious to the surgeon.

breast, or if you tend to have multiple large cysts, this again may be an increased risk factor.

Apart from all the above factors, there is an increased interest in the amount of fat in our diet. Many authorities consider that maintaining a stable, normal weight, and eating a diet relatively low in animal fats and high in fresh fruits, fresh vegetables and cereals may decrease your chances of developing breast cancer.

It has been noted that many women who have had their babies early — and certainly those who have breast-fed for a long time — seem to be much less at risk than women who have had their children late and did not breast-feed.

The current controversy over whether or not the taking of oral contraceptives increases the likelihood of breast cancer is still an open question. The actual effects of oral contraceptives are complicated by the fact that women who have been taking them for a long time tend also to be those who defer their families until later, and it will be some time yet before the specialists can be absolutely clear about whether or not oral contraceptives can increase the risk of breast cancer. At the moment, the majority of studies have produced very little evidence that oral contraceptives cause an increase

DETERMINING YOUR OPTIONS: A LOGIC TREE

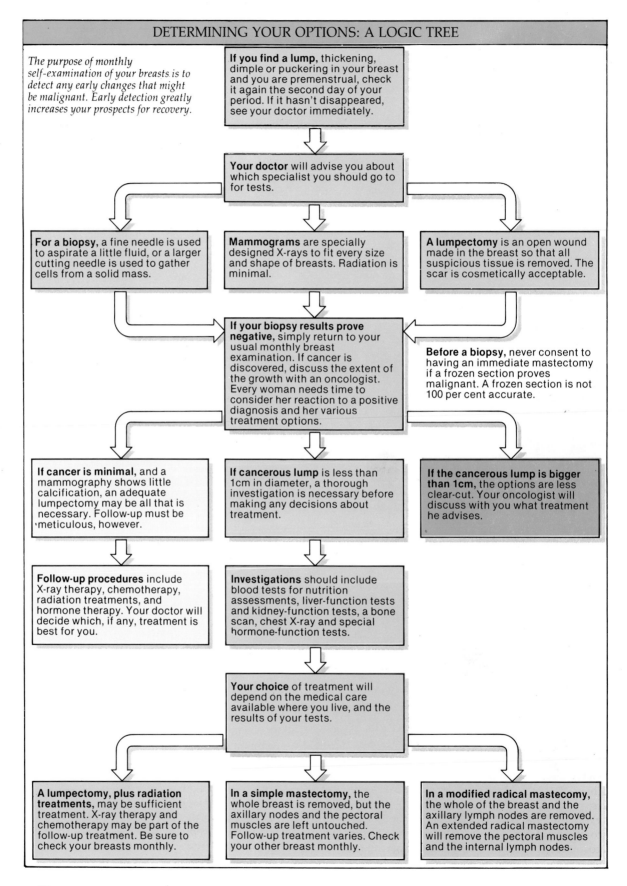

The purpose of monthly self-examination of your breasts is to detect any early changes that might be malignant. Early detection greatly increases your prospects for recovery.

If you find a lump, thickening, dimple or puckering in your breast and you are premenstrual, check it again the second day of your period. If it hasn't disappeared, see your doctor immediately.

Your doctor will advise you about which specialist you should go to for tests.

For a biopsy, a fine needle is used to aspirate a little fluid, or a larger cutting needle is used to gather cells from a solid mass.

Mammograms are specially designed X-rays to fit every size and shape of breasts. Radiation is minimal.

A lumpectomy is an open wound made in the breast so that all suspicious tissue is removed. The scar is cosmetically acceptable.

If your biopsy results prove negative, simply return to your usual monthly breast examination. If cancer is discovered, discuss the extent of the growth with an oncologist. Every woman needs time to consider her reaction to a positive diagnosis and her various treatment options.

Before a biopsy, never consent to having an immediate mastectomy if a frozen section proves malignant. A frozen section is not 100 per cent accurate.

If cancer is minimal, and a mammography shows little calcification, an adequate lumpectomy may be all that is necessary. Follow-up must be meticulous, however.

If cancerous lump is less than 1cm in diameter, a thorough investigation is necessary before making any decisions about treatment.

If the cancerous lump is bigger than 1cm, the options are less clear-cut. Your oncologist will discuss with you what treatment he advises.

Follow-up procedures include X-ray therapy, chemotherapy, radiation treatments, and hormone therapy. Your doctor will decide which, if any, treatment is best for you.

Investigations should include blood tests for nutrition assessments, liver-function tests and kidney-function tests, a bone scan, chest X-ray and special hormone-function tests.

Your choice of treatment will depend on the medical care available where you live, and the results of your tests.

A lumpectomy, plus radiation treatments, may be sufficient treatment. X-ray therapy and chemotherapy may be part of the follow-up treatment. Be sure to check your breasts monthly.

In a simple mastectomy, the whole breast is removed, but the axillary nodes and the pectoral muscles are left untouched. Follow-up treatment varies. Check your other breast monthly.

In a modified radical mastecomy, the whole of the breast and the axillary lymph nodes are removed. An extended radical mastectomy will remove the pectoral muscles and the internal lymph nodes.

in breast cancer, and in some studies they actually seem to have both an ameliorating effect not only on breast cancer but on other breast disorders.

Side effects of breast surgery   The side effects are different for each woman. After a mastectomy, the sensation is very commonly as though the breast is still there. Indeed the feeling may be so strong that you actually feel compelled to touch the breast — only to realize, of course, that it has gone. This curious feeling, called causalgia, or phantom pain, is due to the disturbance at the nerve endings where they have been cut during surgery.

Getting used to being without a breast takes some time; if you have a very heavy bosom, you will feel particularly lopsided and uneven. It is therefore essential for each woman to consider what she can do for herself and be aware of what help she can obtain in order to return to normal as quickly as she possibly can.

Physiotherapy can minimize the effects of muscle loss on the ability to breathe efficiently or move the arm. These exercises usually begin about five days after surgery and they are designed to strengthen the muscles of the arm that will do the job of the pectoral which has been removed; they also play an important part in stimulating the circulation of blood and lymph through the wound, therefore promoting healing.

A prosthesis (a realistically-shaped artificial breast) can be fitted. Usually it is made of silicone, but a variety of prostheses are now available and the options will be discussed with you. The prosthesis of your choice can then be fitted so as to match your other breast. Worn inside your bra, it is completely undetectable when you are dressed.

If the cancerous growth was slight, but a total mastectomy was carried out, some surgeons are now prepared to leave sufficient skin for a silicone prothesis to be fitted underneath, although this is usually not implanted until some time after initial surgery. If beforehand you feel that breast removal would be a particularly traumatic experience for you, it is well worth checking with your surgeon about the possibility of reconstruction – but the time to discuss this is *before* the surgery is carried out. A flexible breast-shaped sac filled with silicon gel or salt water is inserted between the skin and the rib cage. Surgeons have achieved excellent results by doing an internal breast implant and can actually produce nipples by utilizing a small part of the labia.

Learning to adjust   Most women go through depression and anxiety after breast surgery. And a few weeping sessions can actually help you through the inevitable period of adjustment, so don't struggle to suppress them. They are normal and to be expected. But if your experience of depression is severe, you can contact the Mastectomy Association in London (see pages 202/3). Their members, who have had mastectomies, have learned to come to terms with the fact and are leading well-adjusted, normal lives. They will visit you in hospital or at home and be very supportive and reassuring.

The hospital social worker or welfare officer can also organize home help or visits from a health visitor to tide you over the first weeks at home.

Try not to anticipate your partner's reaction to your changed body. Many men actually adjust more quickly than you would imagine. And many are only relieved that the operation has saved your life.

To summarize: all of us are at risk just by virtue of being female and having breasts. Therefore all of us, whether or not we are doctors or Olympic swimmers, must learn to examine ourselves diligently once a month, so that this becomes a lifetime's habit, just like cleaning your teeth. If every woman, from teenager to octogenarian, practised self-examination, then with any luck every cancer could be diagnosed early enough to allow alternatives to surgery to be considered. This practise of 'self-screening' would also be a considerably cost-effective and care-effective change in terms of how we think about breast cancer in the Western world.

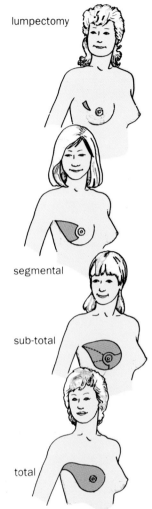

A lumpectomy removes a suspicious area or an early cancer.
A segmental mastectomy removes the whole of the duct system in which the suspicious growth occurs and also removes the nodes associated with that area.
A sub-total mastectomy removes all the suspicious tissue and will usually include a node dissection.
A total mastectomy removes the entire breast tissue and the armpit nodes.
The operation called 'radical mastectomy' — devised over 100 years ago — is still performed in some centres. However, today's techniques of chemotherapy and radiotherapy should mean that it is now only carried out as a last measure.

57

Cervical cancer

In its earliest stage, cervical cancer grows, but does not spread widely. If it can be caught and treated at this stage it can be completely cured. If, however, it progresses further, radical surgery and radiotherapy may be required, and survival is in question. Fortunately, deaths from cervical cancer are decreasing — figures for the United Kingdom in 1983 record 1,959 deaths as against 2,600 for 1981. In younger women, though, the number of new cases appears to be on the increase. For this reason, regular cervical smears (pap smears) are vital.

During cervical cytology, smears from the cervix are taken and subsequently examined under the microscope.
Right: *a slide which shows normal cells. They are neat, clean and regular with clear cytoplasm and a small nucleus.*
Left: *a pre-invasive cancer. The cells look jumbled and have an increased density in their nuclei.*
Right: *an invasive cancer which shows that the architecture of the tissue has broken down and all the cells are completely irregular. The tissue is dense — the cells are tightly packed together and they do not conform to their own spaces.*
In most women the changes from normal cells to pre-invasive (that is pre-cancerous) cells will take many years.

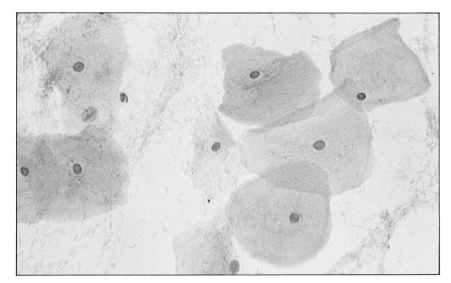

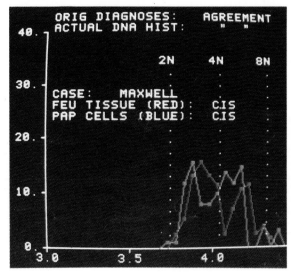

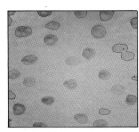

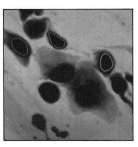

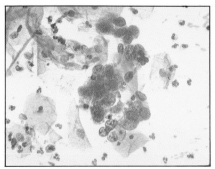

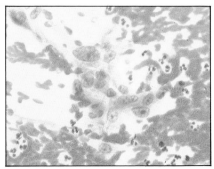

A new development in the analysis of cervical cytology is Automated Cell Diagnosis, in which hundreds of slides can be processed every day at a relatively low cost.
A drop of protein solution is placed on each slide and, if cancerous cells are present, there is a fluorescent reaction. The machine can distinguish between normal cells (above, left) and dyplastic or damaged cells (below, left).
In the computer printout the blue line represents normal cells and the red line abnormal ones, indicating which slides will need the attention of the cytopathologist.

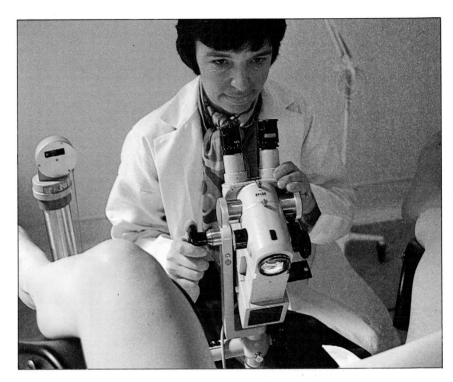

A gyneacologist examines a patient's cervix by looking through a colposcope — a specially designed microscope. This method makes possible the diagnosis of pre-cancerous lesions of the cervix, which sometimes appear as areas of heaped-up tissue.

If the lesions are truly pre-cancerous they can either be treated by cryo-surgery (freezing) or hot cauterization (burning), or by means of vaporization with a laser beam. These treatments remove the malignant cells and possibly the viral, or other, agent which is triggering the changes.

While treatment of early lesions will prevent life-threatening cancer, any woman who has received such treatment must make sure that she attends for a cervical smear every year for the rest of her life.

Tests for cervical cancer   Every woman over the age of 30 should protect herself by having a cervical smear test at least every two years. The whole procedure takes a matter of minutes and is absolutely painless. The results will be notified to your doctor within four to seven weeks (much earlier if they are positive, in which case you will be one of the lucky ones who receive treatment in good time).

Sometimes a woman is called back for a second test. If this happens to you, don't panic. It may simply be that the first smears left an element of doubt because they were, for instance, taken too close to your period — either just before, or just after when some slight bleeding may still be in evidence.

If the tests are positive, a colposcopy is likely to be performed. This is a simple procedure whereby the cervix is examined with the aid of a low-power microscope, enabling a skilled doctor to recognize any abnormality and to take small specimens from suspect areas for further examination. It is completely painless and can be done without the need for an anaesthetic.

Once the results of this examination are known, it may be necessary for a cone biopsy (a means of obtaining an actual piece of tissue from the suspect area) to be made in order to establish the full extent of cancer invasion. A cone biopsy is the *only* way to establish the extent of spread to the internal opening of the cervix. However, you should be aware that the resulting scarring of the cervix may cause problems during delivery in future pregnancies, and that a biopsy in itself can cause pain and bleeding. In larger cities, the use of a laser (available in some hospitals) has proved to be even more effective as a preventative treatment in recent years.

Symptoms of cervical cancer
Cervical cancer has few symptoms and very often they do not appear; this makes the regular smear test even more vital. The most common symptoms of this particular cancer are:
● Bleeding between periods or after intercourse; also post-menopausal bleeding after monthly periods have ceased.
● A watery, blood-stained discharge.

Treatment of cervical cancer

There are two possible treatments: either surgery or radiotherapy, or a combination of both may be used — depending on the hospital giving the treatment and the clinical stage of the cancer.

If a cone biopsy entirely removes the cancer it may be decided to defer further treatment and to carry out regular smear tests to monitor the situation. Much depends on the attitude of the hospital at which you are treated. However low you may be feeling, try to discuss the matter with your surgeon, and if there are any options, make sure that you know what they are.

Ovarian cancer

The early stages of ovarian cancer could be mistaken for early pregnancy as the disease has a similar effect on the gut as the pregnancy hormones.

Symptoms of ovarian cancer

- Any unusual pain or bleeding.
- Change in sexual response.
- Any unusual nausea or indigestion.
- Any increase in size of the abdomen.
- When very large, increased frequency of urination, varicose veins and swollen ankles.

Treatment of ovarian cancer

If, upon examination, your doctor feels a lump in your abdomen or pelvis he or she will refer you for diagnostic ultrasound tests, laparoscopy and, possibly, surgery. Many surgeons favour complete removal of the tumour straight away so, before you undergo any surgical investigation, discuss the options with the surgeon.

Any ovarian cancer means that you will have to have both ovaries removed, no matter what age you are; no doctor can take the risk of leaving ovarian tissue in your body. Differing hospital departments do have varying protocols for treating this disease.

Uterine cancer

The vast majority of women who have uterine cancer are in the fifty-plus age group — its incidence increases sharply with age. Uterine cancer may occur in women who have had little or no sexual activity, and in women who have not experienced childbirth. Other risk factors are thought to be:

- Gross overweight.
- Diabetes.
- High blood pressure.
- Uterine fibroids.
- A family history of uterine cancer.

Symptoms of uterine cancer

- Abnormal bleeding from the vagina, ranging from spotting to heavy, prolonged haemorrhage. Bleeding may also occur after intercourse.
- Cramp-like pains and general pelvic discomfort.
- A need to empty the bladder with increased frequency.

Any woman reporting these symptoms should be given a D&C and if there are cancerous cells, they will be discovered when the scrapings are examined.

Treatment of uterine cancer

- Total hysterectomy and, almost always, radiotherapy.
- High-dose progesterone therapy may be given instead if the disease has already spread to the pelvis and beyond.

As with breast and cervical cancer, the chances of recovery depend on the stage and extent of the disease. So, if any of the symptoms described above occur, go to see your doctor without delay.

Ovarian cancer tends to be a 'silent disease' with few symptoms; if a patient is not referred for diagnostic ultrasound and/or laparoscopy at the first suspicious examination then it may only be detected at a late stage — perhaps when it has spread through the ovary into the peritoneal cavity.

Every woman — particularly after the age of 40 — who experiences any episode of abnormal bleeding, changes in her sex life or appetite, or recurrent episodes of nausea, should have a thorough examination which includes ultrasound x-rays of the ovaries and referral for further consultation if necessary.

Below: it is sensible for a woman to have an annual pelvic examination.

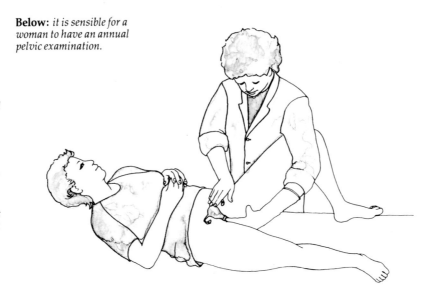

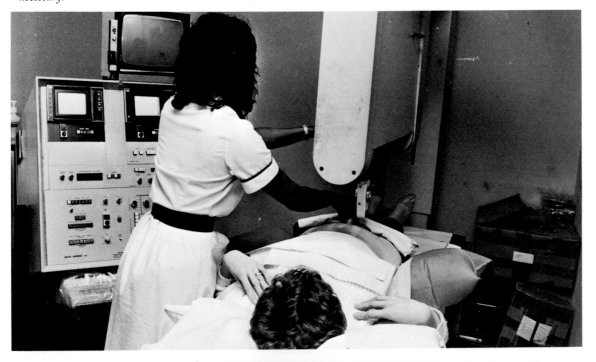

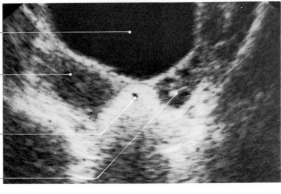

full bladder

cystic ovary

uterus

normal ovary

Pelvic ultrasound is a non-invasive test to examine the anatomy of the pelvic organs. Two hours before the test the patient must drink two pints of fluid; her full bladder will then reflect the sound waves, improving the quality of the x-ray. The resulting pictures will indicate any abnormality in the uterus, Fallopian tubes or ovaries.

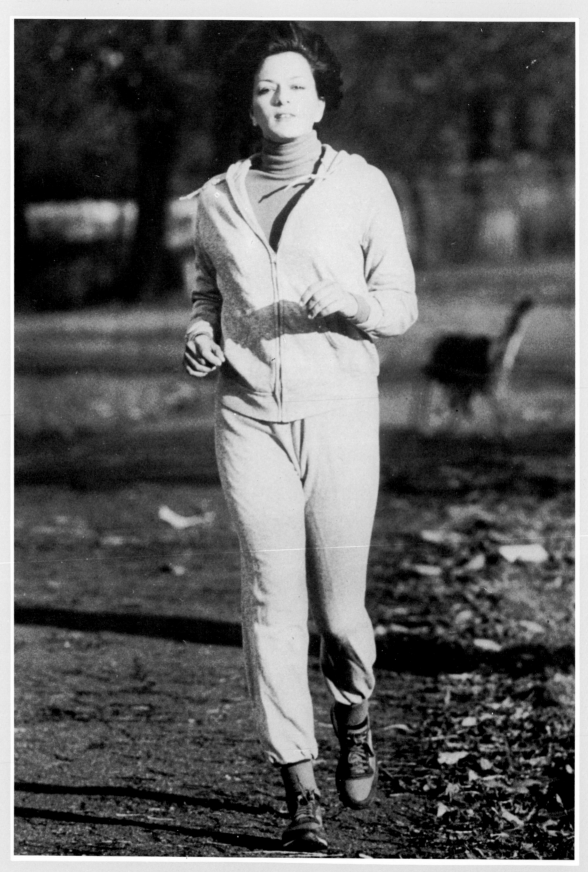

Health Cultivation

● Positive Health ● Images of Women ● Why Dieting does not Work
● The Good Food Guide ● Exercise and Fitness
● Care of the Hair, Eyes, Ears and Teeth
● Emotional and Mental Well-Being ● Relaxation ●

Positive health

Positive health has a particular relevance to women. The following statistics show that on average women live longer than men and at some time of their lives will spend an extended period alone.

Families are getting smaller. The average number of people per household has fallen in the last 20 years, due to a declining birthrate and a steady increase in the proportion of people living by themselves.

Approximately two million women in Britain live alone or spend many hours per day with only small children for company.

Divorce rates have increased five-fold in the last 20 years.

In 1981 the average life expectancy for a man was 69, for a woman 75.

About one third of elderly people in Britain live alone.

More than half of all women aged 75 and over live alone.

Positive health involves becoming aware of and paying attention to every aspect of our lives and in fulfilling the potential within each one of us. It also involves being adaptable. Remaining healthy and in harmony with our constantly changing environment depends on our ability to change and adapt to new situations and people, shifting economic, political and social values. Resistance to change, or ignorance and confusion in the face of change, creates tension and rigidity, insecurity and anxiety – the starting points of illness. So health is not something that resides in the individual alone. Our interdependency with our environment and with other people is experienced most when things either go very wrong, as in serious illness, or are very right, when the harmony we feel in our surroundings and our relationships gives us an inner peace. A consciousness of the whole being – mind, body and spirit – as part of a greater whole – relationships, family and environment – is the essence of holistic health, see page 45. It means being aware of the continuous flow between desires, thoughts, needs and hopes, and the realities, demands, approaches, assistance and cooperation of others.

Positive health also involves being able to alter our environment, just as we can learn to change our inner world through understanding and awareness. This means developing a sense of one's individuality, of taking responsibility for oneself and one's needs, making decisions and choices. It also means developing the capacity to understand and share with others — to know for instance, when it is right to be responsible for someone else, a young daughter perhaps, and to know when to let the child take charge for herself. Or, with another adult, to know when to let go and let him or her take care of you for a while — the development of mutual responsibility.

To aim for positive health rather than an absence of ill-health involves learning to listen to our bodies' language, to the finely tuned rhythms within us which can tell us about ourselves and our state of health. This growing awareness can sometimes be painful; you may become conscious of needs or feelings you have suppressed and of ways in which you hold yourself back from living fully, the fears and anxieties which keep you tied to limiting habits. But awareness brings with it a greater joy too. Pleasures can be felt more keenly, opportunities grasped more confidently, choices made more clearly. Positive health is the full creative potential of each one of us; it is a state of being, a continuous changing flow, an adventure in which we seek a richer and more satisfying way of life.

Taking Stock

The first step towards positive health cultivation is to take stock. Give yourself time to look carefully at your present life, your habits, likes and dislikes, immediate goals, long-term aims and, of course, at your potential for change. Otherwise, any changes you make to your lifestyle and eating habits may well be impulsive and unrealistic. New resolves of this kind are all too easily broken because they may jar with your present lifestyle and involve considerable extra effort.

The second important thing is to take things *slowly* because all change, for better or worse, may cause stress. A marriage, a new lover or job, moving house, or having a baby can all cause anxiety. This is also true of positive changes such as taking up an exercise regime or changing your eating habits. By being too radical or ambitious, people defeat themselves; the daily run or the eating of wholefoods can quickly become just one more burden, another pressure on already highly pressured lives.

This is not what positive health is all about. So take it step-by-step, and remember that progress does not automatically follow a straight and smooth upward curve. There will be times when you feel fed up, when you revert to old ways; there will be periods when you feel no different to the way you were before you took up exercise, started to eat healthily and cut down on smoking or drinking alcohol. Be kind to yourself; old habits are hard to kick, and new ones, however well-intentioned, take a surprisingly long time to establish as an automatic part of your life. Don't make 'getting healthy' into a stick to beat yourself with every time you feel lazy or indulge yourself.

First steps

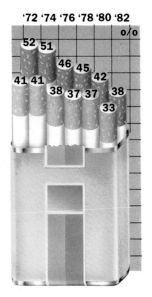

'72 '74 '76 '78 '80 '82

men
women

Men still smoke in greater numbers than women but they have been more successful in giving up — between 1972 and 1982 the proportion of adult male smokers in the population fell by more than a quarter.

Between 1980/82 the percentage of female smokers fell from 37 to 33 per cent. Overall, in these years, more than one million people gave up smoking.

Taking a cool look at how you live may well reveal very obvious problem areas which must be tackled as a first step towards positive health. Making changes will be a great boost to your self-confidence.

Smoking Everyone now should know that smoking causes bronchitis and lung cancer, is a contributory factor to heart disease, is very detrimental to health and fitness generally, and decreases the ability to take in and metabolize oxygen. Yet women are not abandoning smoking in the same numbers as men, and deaths from lung cancer in women are rising. Women's dependence on cigarettes can be attributed to a number of factors, among them the increased independence of women which causes them to acquire the social habits associated with more powerful social and financial positions. There is, too, the increased stress placed on women today, when many are filling several demanding roles simultaneously. Much cigarette advertising is now directed at women, playing on their insecurity in recently acquired positions of responsibility at work and the universal desire for escape into a world of glamour and ease.

Other effects of smoking are that, like all toxins ingested (coffee, alcohol, drugs, sugar, and so on) they use up the body's B and C vitamins (see page 110). Of particular importance to women is smoking's implication in low birth-weight and possible fetal weaknesses; underweight babies have a significantly reduced chance of surviving the first few weeks of life.

If you have real difficulty in giving up there are a number of strategies to help you. A nicotine-based chewing gum has proved very helpful in getting over the worst pangs of nicotine dependency; it is available from a doctor on a private prescription. Anti-smoking classes and other forms of therapy can also be very helpful. You can get in touch with Action on Smoking and Health (ASH) or your local health education unit for information on these.

Alcohol Like smoking, alcohol is a social drug and as such very difficult to avoid, perhaps even more so than cigarettes, in that almost every social occasion begins with the invitation to 'have a drink'. Again, advertisers and manufacturers are aiming their campaigns more at the increasing female market and, just as with smoking, the figures for women with drinking problems are on the rise. The increasing incidence of alcoholism among women is causing great concern in the medical profession.

64

Some nutritionists and doctors think that a moderate amount of alcohol per day — say a couple of glasses of wine or their equivalent — can be beneficial in its relaxing effect, its aid to the digestion, and because it stimulates the production of prostaglandin E1 (needed for the functioning of the immune system). Any more than this moderate amount, however, will have a generally depressive effect. Alcohol depletes the body of B and C vitamins, thus potentially causing depression, fatigue, digestive disorders, cirrhosis of the liver, ulcers and impairment of the circulation. Like sugar, alcohol supplies the body with 'empty' calories, and so contributes to the problems of being overweight. For women, high alcohol consumption during pregnancy contributes to low birth-weight and neural tube defects in the new-born baby.

Fruit juices are preferable to alcohol, especially after diluting them half and half with water to lower their sugar content; try to avoid cola drinks which are entirely composed of sugar.

Body shape has always been a preoccupation in the West and the current obsession is with being thin or getting thin. The whole area of slimming and dieting is of particular relevance to women, for it is they, far more than men, who feel bound to subscribe to the slim ideal, and they, more than men, who diet, buy slimming aids and go on one gruelling slimming regime after another. But although dieting can be considered a specifically female obsession, and one that has perhaps got out of hand, it is also true that obesity *is* a major problem in twentieth-century society. Furthermore, the food we eat has been cited as the single greatest cause of the so-called Western diseases: heart trouble, digestive and intestinal problems, cancers, diabetes, arthritis and rheumatism. All these have now reached epidemic levels.

'You can never be too thin...'

It is clear that the whole issue of fat and thin is an important one both for women and their families. We need to look closely at the problem in order to gain a proper understanding of a subject that preoccupies most women and, increasingly, has come to concern the medical profession. We need to look at why we want to be thin, how thin we want to become, the methods we use to achieve this and whether we are using our energies to pursue an illusion. Most importantly, we need to understand more about the food we eat and, if necessary, to change our eating habits for a healthier life.

Every individual's body has its natural weight, shape and inherent beauty. However, many of us abuse our bodies over the years through bad eating habits, sedentary lifestyles, cigarettes, alcohol and drugs. Consequently, we soon lose that natural beauty, becoming overweight and lacking in energy, with poor health, skin and poor hair. The intention in this section is not to provide you with slimming tips or magic diets to follow blindly in the hope of losing unwanted inches and pounds. The aim of every woman who starts to pay attention to her diet, her weight and her health should be to find the *right* shape and weight for *her*, not to strive for an arbitrary 'ideal' set up by some outside authority. Once you understand the principles of good food and exercise — the two key elements of the energy balance — then you will naturally achieve your proper shape and weight. For many this will involve losing some pounds, for others it may well mean gaining some in the form of firmer muscle.

Fear of fat Studies conducted here and in the United States over the past three decades show that we judge fat women harshly in the West. Whereas the fat man still carries a jolly or powerful image (for instance Father Christmas or Winston Churchill), fat women are seen as unattractive and pathetic. This attitude is inculcated from a very early age. In a 1978 study, conducted by researchers at the Clinic for Eating Disorders at Cincinnati College of Medicine, pre-school children were shown a fat and a thin doll. Ninety-one per cent of the children preferred the thin doll, including those children who

65

were themselves fat and knew that they were so. In further tests the children ascribed mostly negative attributes to the fat doll. Other studies have shown that fat girls are discriminated against in a variety of situations, from competing for university places to shopping in the supermarket.

Most women are acutely aware of the social unacceptability of being overweight and, to avoid this stigma, spend enormous amounts of time, energy and *angst* on keeping themselves from the dreadful fate of fatness. But our fear of flesh has sent us over the top. When 500 people in San Francisco were asked what they feared most, the choice of 190 of them was not nuclear war, unemployment or violent crime, but getting fat. And the Royal College of Physicians in their 1983 report on obesity estimated that 65 per cent of British women are on a diet at any one time. Compare this figure with the findings of a popular survey done in August 1983 in an American woman's magazine: 75 per cent of the women who replied felt that they were too fat and nearly half were moderately or very unhappy with their bodies — this despite the fact that according to the weight tables only 25 per cent of them actually were overweight. The desire to be thin is evidently a powerful one and not always related to reality. And it is not just Americans who are narcissistic: in England, a national opinion poll conducted in spring 1984 showed that one quarter of already slim women — and an even higher proportion of the very thin — wanted to shed yet more pounds. It has now become clear that, in addition to the two per cent of women who are clinically anorexic (and anorexia nervosa is widely known as the 'slimming disease'), many more women are indeed 'in an anorexic state of mind'.

What is meant by 'overweight'? A great many women imagine they are overweight, and equate fatness with being ugly and therefore socially unacceptable. Being fat, they feel, puts them on the margins of society and makes them unloveable. But of those women who are overweight, how many consider the health aspects of being overweight? A *Which?* survey found that out of 1,001 people 58 per cent of the women wanted to slim for cosmetic reasons (as opposed to only 19 per cent of the men), whereas only 39 per cent of the women wanted to slim for health reasons (as opposed to 76 per cent of the men). This is important, because recent findings show that one in four women *need* to lose some weight for their health.

To know whether we belong to that 25 per cent who need to lose weight for health reasons, we need to be clear on what exactly constitutes being overweight. Early weight tables, compiled by American life assurance companies and established on highly unscientific data, have since been found to be inaccurate and are now redundant. They tended to set ideal weights too low, basing their norm on a selective proportion of the population. New weight tables have now been devised. But rather than here provide an essentially arbitrary ideal weight for you to aim for, it is much more helpful to demonstrate a difference between *overweight* and *overfat*.

Every woman, if she is honest with herself, knows when she is putting on weight, knows what it feels like to be the 'right' weight for her, and knows what it is like to feel fat. Because muscle weighs more than fat, a large, sturdily built woman weighs more than a smaller-framed woman of the same height. Yet that lighter woman may well be fatter (in the sense of having too much body fat) than the heavier woman. Weight is relative to, and dependent on, a number of factors: energy consumed, energy given out, frame, height, age, genetic type, lifestyle and metabolism.

The fact is that being underweight, or carrying too little body fat, can be as unhealthy as being overweight or obese. For women, having too little body fat affects their periods, their chances of becoming pregnant and of miscarrying. Statistics show that, for both men and women, being too thin may mean less resistance to disease and infection, fewer resources when fighting illness, deficient nutritional intake, and even risk from heart disease.

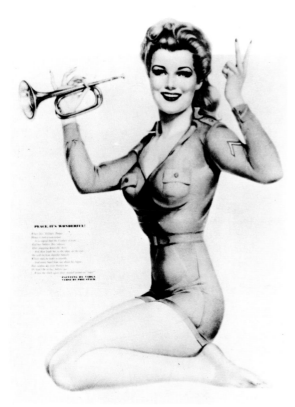

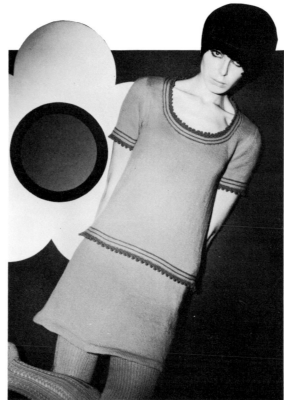

So instead of relying on the scales for guidance, think in terms of shape and the quality of your body tissue. Women often describe their flesh as 'flabby', and although this cruel adjective may sum up a picture of self-hate, it also accurately describes loose, untoned, unused muscle. It is not our weight we should focus on, then, but the health of our bodies. Healthy, firm flesh has a glow and suppleness, the muscles have tone and resilience and the fat is firm and smooth, forming the natural curves and contours of the female shape.

Confusing messages Girls growing up today are exposed to — indeed, bombarded with — conflicting and confusing ideas about what it means to be a woman. We live in a period of great change and transition: more and more women go out to work and are taking positions of responsibility and power. No longer do we automatically consider that a woman's only destiny is to marry as early as possible and to become a stay-at-home wife and mother. Nevertheless, although a great many women now have broader horizons and seek employment or interests outside the home, most women still want to achieve a secure relationship with a man and to have children. These two roles are very often conflicting, and the confusion, anxiety and anger that this dilemma sets up are felt throughout every stratum of society, and by men as well as women. The problems set by the new choices, roles and opportunities open to us, and the new demands made on us, are reflected in our general attitudes to the female shape. The female body is still the chief icon in our culture and is used in advertising to sell everything from cheese to rust remover. Broadly, the types of female bodies admired fall into two categories: the full-busted, 'sexy' woman who features in beer adverts and girlie magazines, and the slender, cool and elegant woman of the diamond and chocolate advertisements. The implicit message of the first image is that she is the earthy, sexually desirable, 'real' woman, appealing to men on a fundamental level, and the second image leaves us in no doubt that here is a successful woman who will be admired and adored as a 'goddess' and who will attract rich and powerful men.

As women we constantly see these stereotyped images and may come to accept them as the norm, yet at the same time recognize that our own shape

Fashions in the female shape change with the times: this svelte but voluptuous blonde — flirtatious but definitely not salacious — allies America's troops from the pages of a 1943 edition of Esquire magazine.

Twenty years later the 'Swinging Sixties' saw a loosening of social attitudes, the emergence of 'Womens Lib', and a look created by such designers as Mary Quant when skinny models — with hollowed faces and jutting collar bones — reigned supreme.

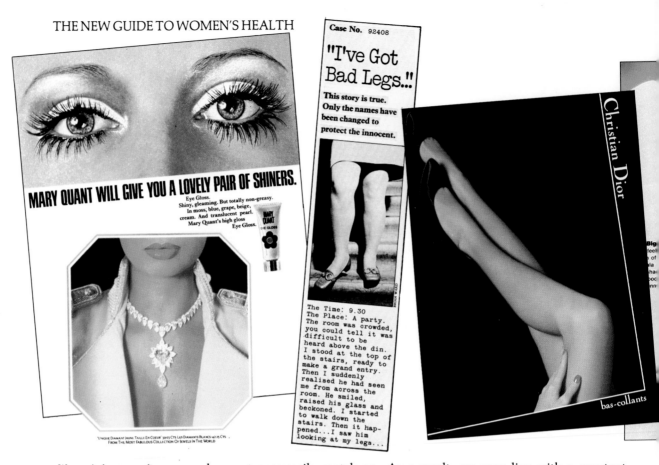

MARY QUANT WILL GIVE YOU A LOVELY PAIR OF SHINERS.

Eye Gloss.
Shiny, gleaming. But totally non-greasy.
In moss, blue, grape, beige,
cream. And translucent pearl.
Mary Quant's high gloss
Eye Gloss.

'Unique Diamant Jaune Taille En Coeur' 39.03 Cts Les Diamants Blancs 147.75 Cts .
From The Most Fabulous Collection Of Jewels In The World

Case No. 92408

"I've Got Bad Legs.."

This story is true. Only the names have been changed to protect the innocent.

The Time: 9.30
The Place: A party.
The room was crowded,
you could tell it was
difficult to be
heard above the din.
I stood at the top of
the stairs, ready to
make a grand entry.
Then I suddenly
realised he had seen
me from across the
room. He smiled,
raised his glass and
beckoned. I started
to walk down the
stairs. Then it hap-
pened...I saw him
looking at my legs...

Christian Dior

bas-collants

Women's faces are often dispensed with entirely in advertising — bits of our bodies being used to sell anything from cosmetics and jewellery to car parts and office equipment.

This fragmentation of the female body not only preys on our own individual insecurities, but also serves to objectify us; the female body is exposed to a kind of prolonged public scrutiny rarely experienced by men.

does not necessarily match up. As a result, we may live with a constant nagging sense of inadequacy.

Advertisements also encourage us to look at our bodies not just as objects but in sections; on one page of a magazine will be a close-up of a girl's hair, on another one of hands, and so on. Men often say things like, 'I'm a legs man, myself,' and women usually complain about specific parts of their bodies: 'It's my thighs, they're so lumpy', or 'I'd be all right if it weren't for my bust.'

Television soap operas encourage similar confusions. The women are mostly slender and glamorous; they are often quite independent and adventurous, but they tend always to be motivated by a man, and eventually to give up their freedom for love. The message all too commonly is: develop your potential, be bright and clever and un-clinging, but this is all in aid of getting a man, and beware of being too brainy or independent or you may intimidate him. No man is ever confronted by such double messages. Our attitudes to ourselves and the way we want to look *are* largely formed by the images we see around us and the standards that our society adopts, so it is important to think about these issues when considering the question of dieting and losing weight.

In the area of food and eating, the double messages continue. On one page of a magazine, for instance, might be a mouth-watering recipe for lemon meringue pie, and on the next the latest tips on how to avoid eating desserts; one section will encourage the cook to concentrate her imagination on preparing delicious meals and another section will be devoted to teaching us how to get thin, how not to indulge in desserts and rich food. Again, becoming aware of this double-think is vital if women want to gain control over their eating habits and their weight.

Food and eating has a particular power for women since it is woman who is the chief nurturer — the first food of life comes from her breast — and it is helpful to become aware of how much time and effort goes into shopping, preparing and cooking food for others and how much energy goes into denying yourself the same nourishment. Having looked at some of the

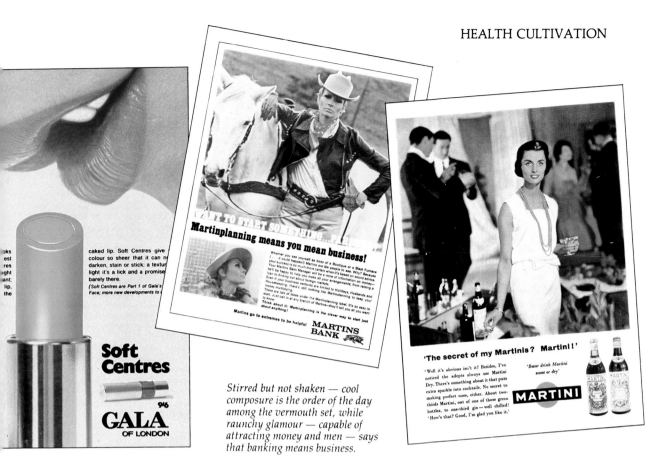

Stirred but not shaken — cool composure is the order of the day among the vermouth set, while raunchy glamour — capable of attracting money and men — says that banking means business.

powerful messages in society which shape our attitudes towards weight and eating habits, we must understand the physical consequences to the whole metabolism of going on a diet.

Why dieting doesn't work   When you go on a low-calorie diet — and all fad slimming diets, from pineapple eating to protein-sparing fasts, restrict calorie intake — your body reacts according to the principle of homoeostasis. Homoeostasis is the body's ability to retain the inner balance of its organs, nervous and digestive systems and blood supply, in the face of a changing environment. The body cannot distinguish between enforced starvation and a crash diet, or between famine and a long-term slimming regime. When you suddenly restrict the body's supply of food, it reacts quickly and efficiently to maintain its inner balance (homoeostasis) and consequently your health.

The first thing that happens   is that you slow down. Studies show that dieters become unconsciously more lazy: they watch more television, take the lift rather than climb stairs, sit around more and generally feel more sluggish. This is your body's way of making sure you use less energy, and is a part of the overall slowing down of your metabolism.

The basal metabolic rate (BMR) — the rate at which your body ticks over — is often assumed to be static. Since the turn of the century, however, research studies have proved this assumption wrong over and over again. Within quite a wide range, our metabolism is very active and volatile. It is affected by physical work, by our emotions, by stress and illness — and by dieting.

Sixty-four per cent of the energy we consume is used by the body's vital organs yet their weight totals only 15 per cent of our body-weight. When you go on a crash diet, the metabolic rate of these vital organs slows down dramatically, by an amount which varies between 10 and 45 per cent of their normal rate. So the less you eat the less energy your body uses.

Over a prolonged period the body adapts to this state of under-nutrition.

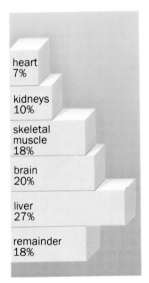

heart
7%

kidneys
10%

skeletal
muscle
18%

brain
20%

liver
27%

remainder
18%

A graphic representation of the percentage of energy used by the body's major systems. Despite all the energy these organs use, they account for little more than ten per cent of the body's actual weight.

WHY DIETING IS BAD FOR YOU

- Dieting slows down the body's Basal Metabolic Rate (BMR); the heart, liver, digestive system, all vital organs and the brain use less energy and function at a lower level of efficiency.
- Your lungs use less oxygen, and therefore all body functions are impaired, particularly the brain. You feel tired, sluggish, listless. Concentration is affected, and some people experience slight dizziness and faintness.
- Dieting affects the delicate fluid balance in the body. Hand in hand with the large amounts of water lost in a diet go many vital minerals, vitamins, enzymes and other hormones. This is called the electrolyte balance. Once this is disturbed, proper reparation of the cells cannot take place, hair and skin growth is arrested, and emotional balance becomes shaky — one of the most frequent comments from dieters is how depressed they feel. Other consequences are anxiety, feelings of hopelessness, panic, pessimism and lack of interest in work and family.
- In the immediate as well as long term, the body's resistance to disease will be weakened by dieting. The body's immune system needs a balanced, daily intake of nutritious food to function properly. Without this you become more vulnerable to viral and bacterial infections and to auto-immune diseases such as arthritis, rheumatism, disorders of the digestive organs, and cancer.
- Psychologically, dieting is a negative, self-restrictive occupation. It is an obsession that uses up energy which could be better spent on creating something good for yourself, on making yourself strong, well, effective and happy. Because of its depressive and weakening physical effects, dieting initiates a downward spiral of self-destructiveness and defeat.

So if you go on a succession of diets, or live on a semi-permanent low-calorie regime, then in effect you train your body to be on a diet. Your metabolism remains permanently lowered and the whole process becomes self-defeating.

The second thing that happens when you go on a low-calorie slimming diet is that you lose weight. Great, you might think; that is just the idea. The diet books tell you that you can lose 10lbs in a week and you assume this to be fat loss. But that is wrong. You cannot lose fat directly in this speedy way, only indirectly; fat stores take much longer to become mobilized for burning as energy. Those 10lbs you lose in a crash diet consist of water and, bound up in the water, glycogen (blood sugar). Glycogen is the body's immediately available source of energy, and it is stored in the muscles and other vital organs. It is essential to the body — providing the instant energy required for all action (from running to catch a bus to lifting a teacup) — and it is the brain's food. The body must replace glycogen quickly once it is lost, particularly after intense effort, illness or a crash diet. Hence the cravings, thirst and disturbed eating habits such as the ravenous hunger and gorging which often force a dieter to break her diet after about 10 days. The body is protecting itself by responding to the altered blood sugar levels; when they fall too low the appestat (the hunger control centre in the brain) is triggered and you feel hungry.

After a while on a low-calorie diet, and once the body has used enough of its immediate source of energy, glycogen, you will start burning fat. The timing of this varies from person to person. However, the body will take its energy and nutrients from the best sources within itself and so will break down lean tissue as well as fat. This is particularly true of a sedentary person whose lean tissue (muscles and organs) are not active and lively. In a particularly strict diet or fast the weight you will lose will be about 65 per cent lean tissue and only about 35 per cent fat.

When you stop dieting and return to 'normal' eating, your body will first replace the glycogen and water as quickly as possible, and then its 'food stores'. If you are a sedentary person your body has no great need for a lot of lean tissue (muscles burn more calories than fat, and therefore need more feeding). So the body will replace the lost weight with fat rather than with lean tissue. And, just as certain training regimes can develop the body to excel in sport, so dieting is a form of training your body — to expect and cope with, as efficiently as possible, food shortage. Fat is the equivalent of the camel's hump; it satisfies the body-needs in times of famine. In this way, dieting can eventually make you fat.

The good food guide

If dieting to stay slim is not the way to good health, then what is? What and how much should we be eating? Nutrition is a young science and still fraught with controversy. However, leading figures in the field are agreed on two fundamental points: the damage that our present diet is doing to us and the need for clearer guidelines towards healthy eating. Some call it the 'new nutrition'. In fact there is nothing very new or complicated about it. In essence it is a diet based on wholegrains, vegetables and fruit, with small amounts of meat and dairy products forming the complement to a meal rather than being its basis. The idea is to eat fresh wholefood and avoid or restrict the intake of fats, refined sugar, white flour, red meat and processed foods containing chemical additives.

The message is essentially a simple one, but, in actuality, changing our eating habits is not quite so easy: it requires a conscious and constant effort. Eating habits are ingrained from childhood and carry all sorts of emotional connotations (few people eat in response to hunger alone) so it usually takes more than just a simple decision to 'eat better' for new habits to become part of one's life. Furthermore, do not underestimate the importance of making changes in the kind of food you eat. The general level of chronic poor health is so widespread that it has become accepted and a lot of people have forgotten what it is like to feel really well and active.

Changing to a wholefood way of eating, with lots of fresh food, can lead to radical and speedy improvements in your health and vitality, and this in turn can benefit every other area of your life. Although you may not realize it until later, the changes you make towards eating well and becoming active could well be among the most decisive, positive steps that you ever take for yourself.

To understand why we need to change our eating habits and give up those cream cakes, rich sauces and quick and easy convenience foods, let's take a brief look at the harmful effects of many twentieth-century foods.

Calorie-dense and nutritionally poor food

When we talk of a food being calorie-dense we mean it is high in calories. A calorie (or more correctly kilocalorie) is a measure of the amount of energy or heat given off when metabolized (or burnt) by the body. The body needs six nutrients: water, proteins, fats, carbohydrates, vitamins and minerals.

Increasingly, the manufacturing industries are refining, preserving and packaging more and more foods. In the process they have created food that is energy-dense but nutritionally poor — foods high in calories and low in goodness. Sugar, fats and white flour have all been refined and treated to remove the perishable substances. It is these living parts, such as the wheatgerm in wheat, that contain the goodness, and after their removal what is left is a product that is pliable, durable, bland, versatile and consistent — all ideal qualities for a process of manufacture which involves machines and keeping foods packaged for great lengths of time on supermarket shelves. But refined sugar, refined flour and commercial fats are dead substances, containing nothing but calories.

As Western nations have become richer their eating habits have become more 'sophisticated'. As a result the food industry has grown to produce more and more 'new lines' to which include chemical additives, preservatives and colouring agents to ensure products of standard flavour and long life, and which are bright enough to attract the eye.

In the early days of nutrition study, attention focused on getting enough of the most well known nutrients — proteins, fats and carbohydrates, and water. This was a relatively easy idea to grasp because they could be identified with specific foods. Thus we were encouraged to eat plenty of meat, milk, butter and other dairy foods for our protein and fat requirements, and bread, potatoes and sugar for carbohydrates. And so the average diet in the West has focused more and more on these foods, including plenty of packaged, canned, and frozen items. Fresh vegetables and fruit, wholegrains, beans and pulses have, to a certain extent, been ignored along with vitamins and minerals.

So what is wrong? We are all aware of the triumphs of modern medicine in combating previously deadly infectious diseases, and because we do not see the grave manifestations of starvation and deficiency diseases, we assume that everyone has enough food to eat and that the general standard of health must be much higher than it was, say, 50 years ago. But in fact, although the general standard of health *is* higher, the incidence of chronic diseases, such as

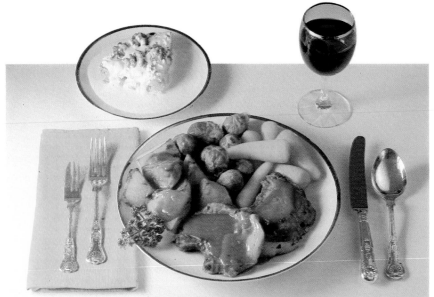

The traditional British meal of meat and two veg, followed by a sugary pudding, is something of a national cliché, conjuring up an image of the comforts of hearth and home. Yet not only is such a meal time-consuming and expensive to produce it is also now widely recognized as actually being a health hazard — high in saturated fats, and with much of the goodness of the vegetables lost in over-cooking.

Burgers, root beer and mass-produced apple pie sum up the 'junk' food that is now available in every high street. By and large these foods live up to the name by which they are known — containing saturated fats, additives and sugar they offer little in terms of nutrition.

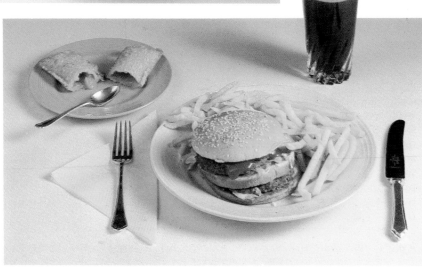

ADDITIVES

May cause digestive disturbance

Causes vitamin B6 deficiency in rats.

May cause reactions in susceptible people: Hay fever, skin rashes etc.

Not permissible on packs in UK.

INGREDIENTS: DRIED VEGETABLES IN VARIABLE PROPORTION (CARROTS, SWEDE, GREEN PEAS, ONIONS, POTATOES, GREEN BEANS, TOMATO, WHEATFLOUR, MODIFIED STARCH (E1422) VEGETABLE FAT, SKIMMED MILK POWDER, SALT, FLAVOURINGS, HYDROLYSED PROTEIN, EMULSIFIER (E450 (c)) COLOURS (E150) (E102) PRESERVATIVE (E220) AND ANTIOXIDANT (E320) (E321)

Raises the lipid and cholesterol levels in the blood.

Linked with possible reproductive failures, behavioural effects, and blood cell changes

Causes irritation of the alimentary food canal

'E numbers' are the key to a list of additives that have been approved for use throughout the European community.

By getting to know what the numbers stand for you can unravel the mystery of what many foods actually contain. E102, for example, stands for a synthetic yellow dye called tartrazine. Many asthmatics are allergic to this substance and it has been implicated in the causes of hyperactivity in children.

The labels (left) list just 12 E numbers; there are, in fact, nearly 300 in use and more are being approved.

Anti-oxidants, pesticides, fungicides, fertilizers, colourants and flavourings, and many more substances, are ordinarily added to the food we eat. There are 3,000 of these additives currently in use, over half of which are cosmetic — that is, used to make the food look plumper or a brighter colour. They are noted on food labels either as E code numbers or under the blanket description 'permitted colourings and preservatives'. The amount of convenience food produced has increased tenfold in the last 30 years.

Chemicals can cause a wide range of adverse effects, but whereas medicines are carefully tested, many additives are not. It costs up to £500,000 to test an additive, and in any case it is difficult to test them conclusively because chemicals added to food are not consumed in prescribed doses like drugs. In addition, what may be a safe intake in small portions of a food may not be so if larger quantities are eaten. There is also the well-known biochemical phenomenon that if you mix two harmless chemicals together you may end up with a harmful concoction. We eat a wide range of modern

foodstuffs today and in unpredicatable amounts. Chemical additives have been cited in the great rise of some cancers in the last few decades; again this is difficult to test because cancers may take up to 20 years to manifest themselves. We do know, however, that many of the additives we ingest are not excreted but are stored in our body-fat, liver and other organs; children are particularly vulnerable, excreting only 50 per cent, whereas adults may eliminate 90 per cent of chemical additives.

Some additives are necessary to preserve processed foods, such as the nitrosamine sodium nitrate in ham which protects us from botulism poisoning; but nitrosamines are simultaneously suspected carcinogens. Vitamin C is used as an antioxidant and may have beneficial effects.

Several additives permitted in Britain are barred by other countries as unsafe. For instance we have 30 artificial food colours in use here, whereas the USA permits ten and the USSR only four. Tartrazine, shown on labels as E102, is a yellow dye put into

buns, sweets and drinks, and is strongly suspected of causing hyperactivity in children and allergies in both children and adults. Some researchers in the US now recommend that we should avoid all food colourings.

Bread contains about 34 additives, among them chlorine gas, used as an oxidizing agent to artificially 'mature' flour, making it stiffer and easier to bake with. It also has the added effect of bleaching it, making for a 'whiter-than-white' loaf.

Pesticides are another example of food additives. Nearly all crops in Britain are sprayed although some of them are banned in the United States. We are all likely to have poisonous pesticides stored in our body fat. This must also be true for livestock fed on sprayed grass and feedstuffs, so the meat we eat is bound to contain some of the chemicals used on the land. This is a major reason for many people's avoidance of meat and the need to wash fruit and vegetables thoroughly.

arthritis, rheumatism, digestive disorders and mental illnesses — is now also much higher. Bacterial infections have given way to the so-called 'degenerative diseases', originally assumed to be a natural consequence of ageing. We now know, conversely, that these diseases are caused not by old age but by Western lifestyles, and particularly by the food we eat. The single major cause of heart disease, arthritis, respiratory complaints, digestive diseases, and 35 per cent of cancers is thus now recognized to be the Western diet — high in refined flour and sugar, fat, red meat and alcohol, but low in vegetables, fruit, wholegrains and cereals, beans and pulses.

Malnutrition — a thing of the past?

We tend to associate the condition of malnutrition with pictures of starving children in Third World countries. The assumption is that here in the West we are better fed than we have ever been. Malnutrition, along with famine, starvation and disease, is a thing of the past, or at least only happens in deprived areas of the world. It comes as a shock then to learn that malnutrition is widespread in the Western world, and that deficiencies are common. The form of malnutrition that we commonly suffer is not due to *lack* of food but to overeating the wrong kinds of foods — those which are 'energy-dense' and 'nutrient-poor' — commonly called 'junk foods' and heavily processed or refined.

However, it is worth remembering that a lot of the 'fresh' food we eat may be partially depleted of nutrients because of long periods of storage in warehouses. Picked before they are ripe, sprayed with chemicals and then left to gather lead pollution in the inner cities, fruit and vegetables cannot be relied on to give us their full complement of nutrients. Additionally, much of the meat we buy is full of growth hormones and antibiotics.

So, unless we are aware of the processes that much of our food is subjected to, and counter this by making sure that our fruit and vegetables are as fresh as possible and that our diet contains a reasonable proportion of wholegrains, beans and pulses, then we are unlikely to get enough nutrients from what we eat. Furthermore, the 'dead' calories we consume — sugar, refined flour and saturated fats, plus toxic additives such as chemical preservatives, colourings, antibiotics and other drugs — actually deplete our body of the nutrients it has stored. This is because the body perceives these dead substances as poisonous to it and marshalls its own resources to deal with them. Caffeine, alcohol, nicotine and other drugs also require the same effort from the body.

Any food that is highly refined has had the vitamins and other elements necessary for its metabolism by the body removed in the processing. So if we eat a diet high in refined foods, drink a lot of alcohol or coffee, smoke, eat processed and sugared foods, white bread and very fatty foods, or live in polluted areas, then we are likely to be experiencing at least mild vitamin deficiencies.

Getting our food priorities right

Healthy eating is simple: no complicated diets or esoteric foods, no tortuous rules or expensive shopping lists. Wholesome, nourishing food is various, interesting and tasty, and lends itself to the lazy cook, to ethnic foods, the eater in a hurry, the gourmet or the lover of fine cuisine. It need not involve learning a whole set of new techniques nor put a further strain on the budget, but it does involve a serious, basic rethink about eating habits and tastes, and discarding some of our favourite prejudices — among them 'Meat and two veg is the only square meal,' or 'A cooked meal is better for you than a cold salad.'

Getting rid of these prejudices is the first step and for some, the hardest. The rest, following the information and guidelines given here, should be an exploration and an enjoyable adventure as you discover for yourself new ways of preparing and eating food. The benefits of adopting simpler, fresher ways of eating are felt by most people immediately. The body responds quickly to the lightening of the load placed on the digestive system, experiencing an increase in energy from slow-burning carbohydrates and the cleansing effects of lots of fresh fruit and vegetables, even if ingrained psychological and emotional attitudes to food are harder to break.

For a woman, it will also have a direct bearing on the well-being of her reproductive and elimination cycles. Most months, a woman's body undergoes hormonal changes even as the demands on her body affect her vitality and emotional well-being. Add to this the stresses and strains of everyday life, which are greater on women today than ever before, and it is evident that we need all the help we can get, and cannot afford to neglect the role of food in determining how we face the world.

The simple process of moving away from quick snacks of sugar- and fat-laden foods towards the foods laid out in these guidelines will have a beneficial effect on your ability to cope with the demands of a busy life. Blood sugar levels will even out, ridding you of those undermining ups and downs of energy and mood. Your sense of emotional and psychological well-being will improve as your body *and* your brain become better nourished.

Many women will also find they lose weight easily and naturally. If a woman needs to lose fat, then her body — given the right assistance — will lose as fast or as slowly as it is ready. Usually, for the body to maintain homoeostasis, fat will be shed slowly. The essence of an approach to food and eating, however, is balance. Some women may well find that their previously undernourished bodies fill out a little, and will need to readjust their self-image along less starved lines and stop abusing themselves with panic crash diets. This is not easy but the increased well-being resulting from these new approaches to eating healthy food will help.

It is much harder to overeat on whole, nourishing foods. And body signals which indicate 'enough' function healthily on unrefined foods. Following this eating plan is one of the very best cures for women who gorge, for bulimics and for those with insatiable cravings. It returns the body to balance. The rewards of eating fresh wholefoods and a high proportion of raw food, fruit and vegetables, are not just an absence of illness or the curing of heart disease and digestive disorders. Eating well is a key part of positive health. This involves giving up the attitude that we have adopted for so long, a mixture of self-deprecation and wanting to please: 'Oh, don't mind me, I eat anything,' towards the attitude that as women we do matter, our health matters, it does matter what we put into our bodies and we do have a choice in what we eat. Caring for ourselves — which includes paying attention to the food we eat — is the prerequisite in caring for others.

A good food guide will not offer diets or recipes but give information and guidelines instead. Eating is a part of every individual's lifestyle and so must be determined by every woman for herself, each taking into account her own cultural and ethnic practices. Also, no two people have the same nutritional requirements; what is indigestible for one person may help another to thrive. Just as no two people have the same fingerprints, so we each have our own food and eating requirements. It is important to be aware of this because it knocks on the head the 'rightness' of social conventions, such as eating at fixed times three times a day.

Since the end of the last century, when the Swiss doctor Max Bircher-Benner 'invented' muesli, and Sir Robert McCarrison conducted his pioneering research in India, the virtues of raw foods over their cooked versions have been explored, researched, studied and, more recently, their health-promoting and curative values widely extolled by some of the most persuasive voices in the current debate about nutrition. These are their main conclusions:
• Cooking destroys many vitamins and minerals, reducing the nutritional and digestive value of food.
• Raw food diets have been found to help in a variety of illnesses, from

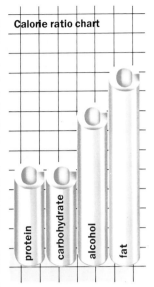

Calorie ratio chart

protein | carbohydrate | alcohol | fat

Fat and alcohol are the most concentrated source of energy or calories, and consequently the most fattening. Fat provides twice as many calories as either carbohydrate or protein.

If you reduce your fat intake — by eating such foods as bread, pasta, fresh fruit and vegetables, rice and cereals — then you not only reduce your calorie intake but also the levels of cholesterol in your blood, decreasing the risk of falling prey to heart disease.

The value of raw foods

digestive disorders to some cancers. They also have a role in preventing heart disease and in convalescence.

- Studies show that people can live very healthily on diets supplying less than the minimum recommended requirements of calories, proteins, fats and carbohydrates, so long as the food they *do* eat is raw.
- Some raw foods, such as muesli, are easier to digest once the muscles of the digestive system have been retrained from a state of laziness due to a soft, undemanding diet of processed foods.
- Raw foods offer a wide variety of tastes and culinary possibilities, and can be inexpensive.

The food balancing act

Of course, we all have to adapt and compromise. Few of us have the time to sit around all day contemplating what we want for our next meal, and no one can prepare individual meals for each member of the family. But if your meals are planned with foods from the groups below in mind, then you should be on the right road to getting your food priorities right.

The basics

Cereals Wholewheat, rye, oats, barley, buckwheat, cracked wheat, millet, brown rice, wholemeal bread, muesli (no sugar), porridge, shredded wheat.
Beans and pulses Chick peas, kidney beans, lentils, split peas, butter beans, mung, aduki, black-eye beans.
Fruit and vegetables Choose a wide variety — roots, tubers and leafy green. The dark, leafy, green vegetables provide a rich source of minerals such as iron. Eat at least one raw salad a day. Buy fresh, lively-looking produce — garden and organically grown vegetables and fruit are particularly valuable because they have not been sprayed.

The complements

Seeds, nuts and eggs Nature concentrates goodness in the reproductive parts of all creatures, so two or three eggs per week plus nuts and seeds added to cereals and salads, are excellent sources of protein and other nutrients.
Sprouts Sprouted grains and seeds greatly increase their vitamin and amino-acid content, so becoming an even better source of protein. They should be eaten fresh and raw, for cooking destroys much of their value.
Milk and live yoghurt These are good sources of protein and other nutrients. Yoghurt is an excellent staple in healthy eating. Delicious in sweet or savoury dishes or eaten on its own, it makes a good substitute for cream, being low in fat and calories and high in protein. Easily assimilated by the body, it encourages the growth of intestinal bacteria called flora which aid digestion. Flora are destroyed by highly acid foods (like coffee, tea, alcohol, sugar and meat), by antibiotics and by other drugs.

To be of nutritional value yoghurt must be 'live' — that is, must contain the beneficial culture or bacteria (indicated on the side of the carton) which aids digestion. The synthetic whipped mixture widely available may taste vaguely similar to yoghurt but there is no comparison nutritionally and it is of no value to health or digestion.

Fish A good source of animal protein and essential minerals and oils. Fish roe, like other 'eggs', are concentrated sources of nourishment. Research indicates that fish protein may have a protective effect against heart disease.

The treats

Meat, poultry, cheese and other dairy products None of these is essential to health, and they are all expensive. Rich in saturated fat, they are a burden to the digestion, the metabolism, the circulation and the kidneys. Since they come at the end of the food chain (from seed, to plant, to animal, to manufacturer, to consumer) they are also likely to retain the chemicals used in their manufacture and processing. Eat them as treats, sparingly.
Wholemeal baking Cakes, biscuits and pastry are all high in fat and many also in sweetness. The sugar content of these occasional treats should be

THE BASICS

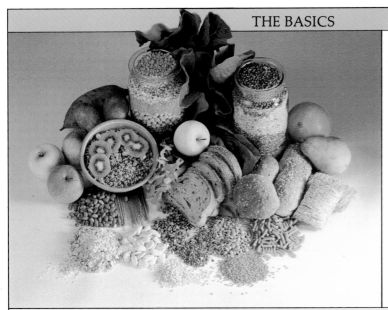

Make sure that a wide range of fruit and vegetables together with beans, pulses and cereals form the basis of your diet. This is the healthiest way of eating and guarantees a low intake of fats and calories yet is high in fibre.

Always make sure that the food is fresh and, if possible, organically grown. Aim to eat as much raw food as possible — at least one salad a day: there are so many quick and easy variations — celery, chopped apples and raisins, for example — that you should not be stuck for inspiration.

Beans and pulses can be used in tasty combinations in salads, casseroles and curries — chilli con carne, dhal (lentil soup or curry), minestrone and humus (chick peas).

THE COMPLEMENTS

Seeds, nuts, eggs, milk, live natural yoghurt and white fish are excellent foods to be eaten in addition to the basics. But some — eggs, for example — are quite rich and should be eaten less often than the others — two to three times a week is ideal.

Nuts, too, complement cereals and pulses particularly well but they are high in fat so be careful not to overdo them. They make interesting additions to salads and add 'bite' to crumble toppings.

White fish can be served grilled or poached, seasoned with lemon and herbs. It provides low fat protein and is delicious when cooked with vegetables in stews and curries.

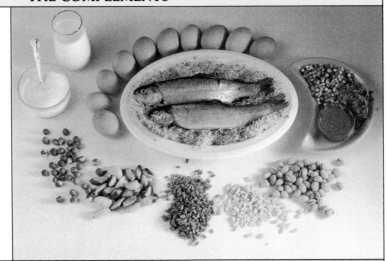

THE TREATS

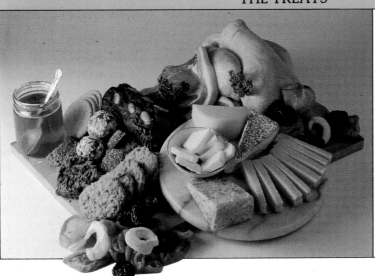

You can still enjoy poultry, red meats, cheeses and other dairy products provided your consumption of them is quite sparing. By cultivating a varied and imaginative wholefood diet, though, you will probably find that your appetite for such rich foods actually decreases.

Poultry is preferable to red meat which you should use only in minimal quantities — in a bolognese sauce with wholemeal pasta, for example, or with aubergines (or potatoes) in moussaka.

Cottage cheese and soft, skimmed milk cheese are good alternatives to the traditional varieties.

SEEDS AND SPROUTS

The seed or egg of any living organism — plant or animal — contains a lot of nourishment. Furthermore, plant seeds are plentiful and cheap compared with other protein sources. Remember that grains in their unprocessed form are also seeds. Less well known is how to grow them, what to do with them, how to eat them, or whether to cook them, sprinkle, grind or munch them. Here are some brief ideas to start you on your way:

• The seeds that are good to eat in their natural state are: poppy, sunflower, sesame and pumpkin. Others are usually cooked or sprouted.

• Combine sesame, sunflower and pumpkin seeds as a delicious, crunchy breakfast

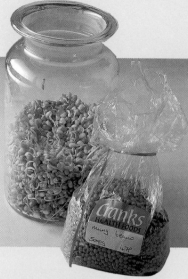

Whole grains and seeds are cheap and nutritious — your local wholefood or health food shop should have a good range to choose from.

topping. Together these three seeds make a complete protein. They are alkaline and provide essential fatty acids, linoleic and linolenic, which are vital to the health and elasticity of

skin and glands, and help to balance cholesterol levels.

• Add sunflower seeds to cooked grain — buckwheat, for example — which already has a warm nutty flavour, for added nourishment and texture.

• Use seeds in crumble toppings and in salads.

• Make up seed, nut and dried food mixes for snacks and children's lunch boxes.

• Use poppy and sesame seeds in bread and other baking.

• All seeds and beans can be sprouted. This increases their nutritional value immensely. Add to salads and sandwiches.

derived from dried fruit or small amounts of honey or molasses (both of which are just as sweet as sugar, and contain trace elements, other minerals and vitamins).

Dried fruit This is a good source of natural, but very concentrated, sweetness. Add to muesli or soak in water for use as a dessert, but do not eat very much in its dried form because the level of sweetness is so high that it will keep alive a craving for sugar. Another good reason for not eating much dried fruit is that most commercial produce is sulphured to keep it looking plump and glossy. Some wholefood stores now sell unsulphured dried fruit which, despite its dull, shrivelled appearance, is worth seeking out and actually tastes better.

Special nutritional requirements for women

Preconception-/early pregnancy

Three to six months before conception you should begin thinking seriously about your diet, especially if you do not usually pay attention to eating regular, balanced meals. The future health of your baby will largely depend on giving your own body good nourishment from a time well before the fertilization of the egg. If you do not, you may actually reduce your chances of conceiving, because the hypothalamus responds to vitamin deficiency by suppressing the release of hormones responsible for fertility. Vitamins A, B_6, and folic acid, and the minerals zinc and magensium are particularly important. Folic acid, a B vitamin, is essential to the manufacture of DNA and RNA, the genetic material of the cell. Zinc, found in leafy green vegetables and wholemeal bread, is the mineral most often mentioned not only in connection with pregnancy but for women generally, particularly since it has now been calculated that a large proportion of the population is deficient in it.

Zinc plays a part in many body processes, among them the absorption of other vitamins and minerals, notably folic acid, and a deficiency of it in pregnant women has been linked with the incidence of spina bifida. The official recommendation is that pregnant women need 20mg daily, but much higher levels, such as 100mg daily, have a curative effect on problems such as skin disorders and water retention. It is found in whole grains, pulses and meat. Zinc and calcium also protect us from the effects of lead pollution. In one study, abnormally high levels of lead in combination with very low levels of zinc and calcium were found in the bones of stillborn babies.

Babies

Healthy eating habits are formed in babyhood; the way you feed your baby is therefore crucial, not only in helping it to grow healthy and strong but in the foundation you lay down for the food choices he or she will make as an adolescent and adult.

Absolutely no salt or sugar should be given to a baby. Choose baby food brands that are salt- and sugar-free and do not add any to the food you prepare for the baby yourself, even if the food seems very bland.

The same nutritional requirements apply to babies as apply to us. If a baby has a small appetite or is fussy about eating, feed him or her often and make the food more energy-dense by adding a little olive (or other high quality polyunsaturated) oil to the food. Do not cultivate a sweet tooth by tempting your baby with sugary confections.

Toddlers

Growing toddlers tend constantly to demand snacks. Give them bananas and dried fruit, but not nuts or raisins as these are one of the major causes of choking in young children. Slices of fresh fruit, sandwiches, very small pieces of cheese, and plain scones are quick and easy and far healthier alternatives to sticky cakes and biscuits. For quick suppers, if you must use convenience foods, serve fish fingers and baked beans rather than any of the preserved, processed or canned meats, such as sausages and spam.

Adolescents

Most adolescents want to eat what their friends are eating, and all go through a period of consuming junk food. Being young and fit and absorbed in the business of living today, they cannot conceive that all those hamburgers, colas, ice creams and white bread are either doing them harm now or will cause them trouble later in life. They do not want to think about such issues and rarely connect their skin and hair problems with unhealthy eating habits. Even when they do become aware of the connection they are often loath to give up the seductive taste of first freedom, eating in cafés with friends, grabbing snacks from take-aways and feasting on 'forbidden foods'. As a mother the best that you can do is to provide wholesome food at home so your child's growing body receives adequate nourishment. If healthy tastes have been cultivated during childhood, the chances are that the taste for junk food will be just a passing phase.

Over-fifties

This is a time when many women lose their husbands; more than half of all women over 75 live alone. No longer cooking for a loved one, there is a tendency to lose interest in food, to become careless about eating properly and to use more convenience and snack foods. Vitamin C deficiency is thus prevalent among older people and scurvy can even occur; if you are in this age group, eat a fresh salad every day and plenty of fresh fruit.

It is important to get enough zinc as bones become increasingly brittle with age due to lowered calcium absorption and zinc assists calcium metabolism. Calcium is also depleted from the body through lack of exercise; exercise is therefore esential in maintaining healthy muscles and bones.

Tiredness caused by lack of adequate nourishment contributes to the apathy many elderly people feel about caring for themselves. The social aspect of eating is important to all of us and particularly in these circumstances. Try to arrange social events involving meals, and share the preparation of the food with friends; this sharing can be as 'nourishing' as the food itself.

Exercise and fitness

For women of all ages, exercise has become one of the most accessible and reliable paths to self-discovery and self-realization. As a woman's body becomes stronger and more effective, so her self-esteem rises. Getting rid of the fragile 'little-me' image and moving from being a spectator to a participant brings new confidence and pleasure.

Research studies into the psychological benefits of exercise show it to be remarkably effective in combating depression, anxiety and other negative and self-destructive emotions. This is of particular relevance to women. They make up the majority of sufferers from psychological disorders (although not from breakdowns).

Exercise encourages women to be assertive, giving them the confidence to stand up for themselves and their opinions. As they become physically stronger and more supple, they feel less physically vulnerable and afraid of harassment. Joggers, particularly, gain a great sense of courage from the thought that if trouble looms they can at least run — and they can probably run faster than most people.

Similarly, as the body's circulation improves and thermogenesis (heat production) increases, so a woman feels less inclined to bundle up against the cold. A great many women find that once they take regular exercise and get used to continuing through rain, snow, slush and heat, get used to feeling sweaty and dirty, get used particularly to the freedom of moving fast and with skill in minimum clothing and flat shoes, unhampered by handbags and high-heeled shoes, so their attitude to the great outdoors changes considerably. In fact, most alter their ways of dressing to accommodate the new sense of freedom they have gained, opting for flatter shoes, fewer layers of clothing, easy-care haircuts and less make-up.

PREVENTATIVE HEALTH CARE

Exercise combined with a healthy diet is the surest preventative medicine and a major component of positive health. Heart disease is still the biggest killer in the United Kingdom, and women are by no means exempt. Exercise is one of the best ways to combat stress and the clogging up of the arteries both of which contribute to heart disease. It is an essential part of a healthy lifestyle. It balances the body and improves its functioning in three different ways:

Fitness   Regular, rhythmic, exercise tones the muscles, increases endurance and stamina, and improves the cardiovascular system, making your heart and lungs stronger.
Strength   Shorter bursts of strenuous exercise strengthen your muscles, making physical work easier. This helps to improve your posture and protect your spine and vital organs, making such common ailments as lower back strain less likely.

Flexibility   Stretching exercises help to keep muscles and joints supple. These, combined with exercises for mobility help to maintain the full range of body movements, preventing the common afflictions of arthritis and rheumatism, and the stiffening up that so often accompanies the process of ageing.

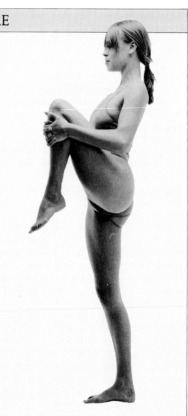

Yoga and dance are both superb forms of exercise; regular practise will bring a deep sense of well-being and relaxation.

When previously non-active people assume a more active life-style, they quickly realize that their tolerance for physical effort is limited. At the beginning, exercise quite literally shakes everything up and provokes varying degrees of physical discomfort. Muscles ache, backs strain, and stomachs swell as the digestive system reacts to the shock of movement. At this stage many people simply give up. There are no visual changes in the body in those first few days or weeks, and what's more it hurts!

Tiredness and stiff muscles the day after are the most common complaints from many newcomers to a regular exercise routine. The main cause is usually 'too much, too often, too soon'. Exercising unused muscles should be a gradual affair with rest days in between. But rest days do not mean sitting at home with your feet up. This merely causes the muscles to contract and tighten, making it feel even harder the next time you exercise. To stop muscles from stiffening the day after, try to be mobile — walk and take the stairs rather than the lift. Take a hot bath immediately after the exercise, then gently massage the muscles. The secret of enjoying exercise is to pace yourself sensibly, increasing gradually.

Preparation   The second most common cause of abandoning exercise is failure to appreciate the importance of warming up and cooling down when doing any strenuous sport. Cold muscles injure easily, and a sleepy body gets a rude shock when suddenly jerked into violent movement. Similarly, if you bring your system to an abrupt halt at the end of a game of squash or a run without a gentle warm down, muscles may go into spasm and the heart may start to palpitate. When exercise ceases, the blood flow to the heart is no longer assisted by the pumping action of the muscles. This causes a build-up of pressure in the muscles which results in an accumulation of waste product fluids (lactic acid). The next day the effect is felt as stiffness and aching muscles. The worst thing you can do after physical exertion is to sit down and flop. See the warm-up and warm-down exercises overleaf for a simple and effective way to get the system going and to keep it gently ticking over before and after exercise.

Attitudes to our bodies   One thing that hinders a lot of women from taking exercise is the fear of stripping off and exposing what they have come to think of as the only female body with lumps and bumps in the world. Western women rarely see each other's bodies in a close and easy intimacy, whereas many men continue some form of sport into middle age, and enjoy the easy camaraderie of the changing room. Surveys show that most women give up sport as soon as they possibly can.

From adolescence onwards, women's bodies change more radically than men's, and the natural confusion and awkwardness that young girls feel with the hormonal happenings in their bodies is compounded by the way in which we feel embarrassed and shy about our bodily functions. The tremendous variety of the female body, instead of being considered by us as something wonderful and exciting, usually provokes insecurity in every woman: 'I don't fit the standard, I don't match up, I'm ugly.' However, although this fear of exposure acts as an initial hindrance to taking up exercise, once a woman does so and sees other women like herself, facing such fears is very liberating. Moreover, with the wonderful range of attractive sports and dance wear now available, exercise can afford as much opportunity for dressing up as going to a party. The timid now have the chance to get fit without the horror of feeling on stage but not dressed for the part.

Sport is unfeminine   In other, possibly less sophisticated societies than ours, it is accepted that women do heavy work and have strong bodies. It is only in the highly-automated societies of the West and in the top echelons of eastern cultures where women are considered to be part of the wonderful array of

What stops us exercising?

WARMING-UP

A warm-up programme is vital before any vigorous exercise and need only take a few minutes. Such a routine is particularly important if you are un-used to strenuous physical exercise — squash, tennis, circuit training or skiing, for example. By warming up and loosening your muscles and getting oxygen into them you will help prevent strains. After your activity you may well ache all over; do not give up as these aches and pains will ease with regular exercise.

The routines shown are good for general fitness too. Breathe deeply and evenly throughout, and perform each movement equally on both sides of your body.

Sit on the floor with the soles of your feet together holding your calves or ankles. Curve your back and bounce your head towards your feet. Stretch your legs out in front

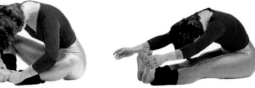

of you. Flex your toes so that your heels are off the floor. Bending forward, stretch out your arms so that your hands are beyond your feet.

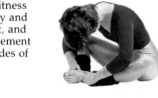

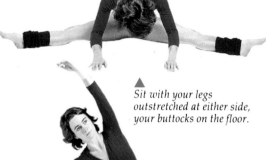

▲ *Sit with your legs outstretched at either side, your buttocks on the floor.*

Curve your spine, stretch out you arms towards your toes and bounce gently.

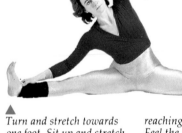

▲ *Turn and stretch towards one foot. Sit up and stretch one arm over the top of your head, your other hand* *reaching towards your foot. Feel the stretch along the whole of your side.*

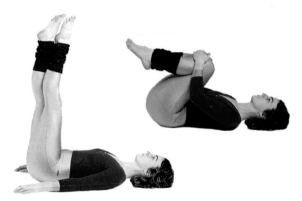

▶ *Kneel with your arms outstretched. Keeping your body in a straight line, lean back gently. Hold for a moment and then return. Repeat as many times as you can. Keep your shoulders relaxed throughout.*

▲ *Lie flat with all parts of your spine on the floor. Lift your legs up at right angles to your body. Criss-cross your legs backwards and forwards in a scissors movement. Slowly lower your legs to the* *floor, criss-crossing them at the same time. Breathe deeply throughout. Bring your knees into your chest to relax your stomach muscles. Breathe deeply then start again.*

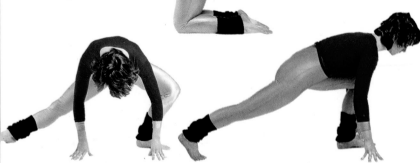

◀ *Crouch down with one leg extended behind, your front foot flat on the floor. Stretch your back heel towards the floor. With your legs in the same position, twist your body to face the front. Bounce towards the floor to stretch your knee and inner thigh. Repeat with your other leg.*

COOLING-DOWN

Cooling down gradually after vigorous exercise is important. Carry out these exercises for a few minutes to give your heart and circulation a chance to slow down. Your breathing should be deep and rhythmic; your muscles should feel warm and relaxed.

After your exercise take a hot shower if possible and dress warmly. Beware of going out into the cold with a sweaty body as you will be vulnerable to chills.

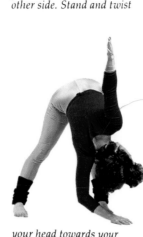

Lift your arms above your head and push them, one at a time, as high as you can reach. Take your right hand down to your left leg. Try to bounce your head towards your left knee. Repeat on the other side. Stand and twist

your upper body first to one side, then to the other. Your arms should be level with your chest.

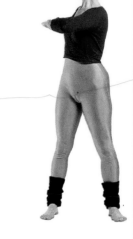

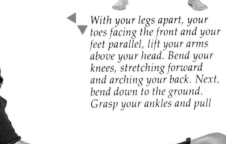

With your legs apart, your toes facing the front and your feet parallel, lift your arms above your head. Bend your knees, stretching forward and arching your back. Next, bend down to the ground. Grasp your ankles and pull

your head towards your knees. Straighten your legs and hold. Release your ankles and slowly uncurl your spine. With your shoulders relaxed, slowly bring your head up to a standing position. Repeat.

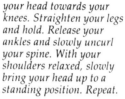

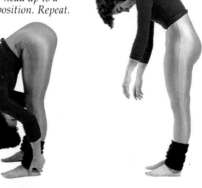

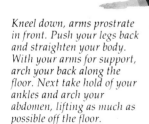

Kneel down, arms prostrate in front. Push your legs back and straighten your body. With your arms for support, arch your back along the floor. Next take hold of your ankles and arch your abdomen, lifting as much as possible off the floor.

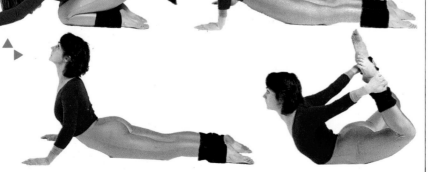

choice consumer goods, that a woman's body must be soft and delectable. Just like chickens which are kept penned so they can't move and put on fat, so women have been discouraged from experiencing their bodies as strong, active and capable of physical exertion.

The time has come to forget all that conditioning and learn from the new images of attractive women who know that beauty comes from whole health which is a result of being fully alive and active, whole individuals who are strong in mind, spirit and body.

Exercise will make me hungry Many women are afraid to take up exercise for fear it will increase their appetite and they will put on weight. In fact, the opposite happens. Women who do regular, strenuous — but not exhausting — exercise report that they do not come home feeling ravenous. On the contrary. There are a number of reasons for this.

Exercise increases your metabolism, the rate at which your body ticks over. The resulting metabolic rate (RMR) is the largest single user of energy, and after strenuous exercise it remains raised by 10 per cent or more for up to 48 hours. When your metabolism functions faster and more efficiently, you feel better in every part of your body: your blood circulation is improved, and movement of bowel and intestines is increased so that food passes through your body more quickly. You also burn more fat from your body stores because your need for oxygen is increased. Using the analogy of a fire in a hearth, it is apparent that the logs (our fat stores) will only begin to burn when they have been set alight with kindling (our blood sugar stores) and the blaze encouraged with bellows (our lungs). When our lungs function more fully we take in more oxygen and burn our food more brightly.

TESTS FOR FITNESS

Before you start an exercise programme test how fit or unfit you are by running on the spot for 30 seconds or do step-ups on to the second step of a staircase for one minute. Afterwards, find your pulse at your wrist or neck (do not use your thumb) and count the number of beats for 15 seconds, then multiply this figure by four. When you exercise, your heart rate should not exceed this rate to begin with. Obviously, as you get fitter your heart will grow stronger and your capacity greater, but your heart rate should never exceed 60-80

per cent of its maximum rate. To find our what your average maximum is, subtract your age from 220. Aim to gradually build up your exercise to a period of at least 15-20 minutes at this heart rate for maximum benefit.

Make sure you do these tests before embarking on *any* exercise regime. If you have tested your fitness as above and your pulse is over 100 beats per minute ten minutes after exercise ceases, or if you suffer from a weight or blood pressure problem, it is advisable to see your doctor for a check-up.

Age	maximum rate (per minute)	60-80% rate (per 15 seconds)	60-80% rate (per minute)
under 25	200	30-40	120-160
25 - 29	195	29-39	117-156
30 - 34	190	28-38	114-152
35 - 39	185	28-37	111-148
40 - 44	180	27-36	108-144
45 - 49	175	26-35	105-140
50 - 54	170	25-34	102-136
55 - 59	165	25-33	99-132
60 - 64	160	24-32	96-128
65 and over	155	23-31	93-124

Grasp your left wrist with your right hand so that you can feel your pulse under your thumb. Then either count the number of beats per minute or count for ten seconds and multiply by six. This figure gives you your pulse rate.

Your choices of exercise

Any kind of exercise is good for you, but for women who want to be fit rather than train as athletes, aerobic exercise is excellent for promoting all round health. Most important is that you choose something you enjoy. Exercise is not a duty and should really be renamed 'play' to banish the puritan image that still lingers in some minds. Just as play is an essential part of a child's growing experience, it is equally important for an adult's sense of well-being. Exercise that is a drudgery, undertaken solely because it is meant to do you good, will not benefit you half as much as exercise that you enjoy. Anything done just for the end result is a heartless activity, and the same goes for exercise.

In deciding which kind of exercise is the one for you, think about the following:
- Do you prefer to exercise alone or with others?
- Would you like the camaraderie of joining a club?
- What time of day do you want to exercise — before breakfast, at lunch-time, after work?
- How regularly can you spare the time?
- How fit are you already?
- Have you done any regular form of exercise before?
- Which kind of exercise best fits your routine?
- Can you afford equipment such as rackets or shoes?
- What about the cost of memberships? Some sports are more expensive than others in terms of initial outlay — club membership fees, etc.
- Do you know the location and opening times of sports centres and facilities near where you live or work?

All these factors will affect your choice of exercise.

Aerobic and anaerobic exercise

Endurance, or aerobic activity, is simply exercise which involves the muscles continuously for a sustained period of time at below maximum effort. Aerobic — literally 'with air' — means exercise which depends on a steady supply of oxygen to maintain the activity for a minimum of ten minutes. This kind of endurance exercise increases stamina by enhancing the ability of the muscles to use oxygen and by improving and strengthening the cardiovascular system.

Aerobics For many people the term 'aerobics' brings to mind the activity of dance and exercise done in a studio to music. These classes have attracted a great deal of criticism due to the large and ever-increasing number of injuries sustained by participants. By association, all exercise classed as 'aerobic' has gained a somewhat confused reputation. However, the two should not be branded together.

Although exercise that falls into the aerobic category (see overleaf) is undoubtedly good for you, aerobics classes, often supervized by teachers with little or no training and even less understanding of the body's anatomy and physiology, can be dangerous. In fact, the very title is a misnomer in that the exercises are mostly *anaerobic* (see below), concentrating largely on exercising each muscle group to maximum effort. Also, the bouncing movements that many teachers practise in these classes are not only counterproductive but may be damaging to the muscles; bouncing damages the fine spindle fibres within the muscle which can't stretch that quickly. If you think of a rubber band (although the muscle is more complicated than this), when you stretch it quickly and then release it, it snaps back to its original state. Muscles should be treated more gently with slow, long stretches which encourage them to relax and become longer without strain.

Anaerobic exercise In these exercises and sports muscles are used to their maximum in a massive effort, the kind of effort that cannot be sustained for

SOME AEROBIC SPORTS

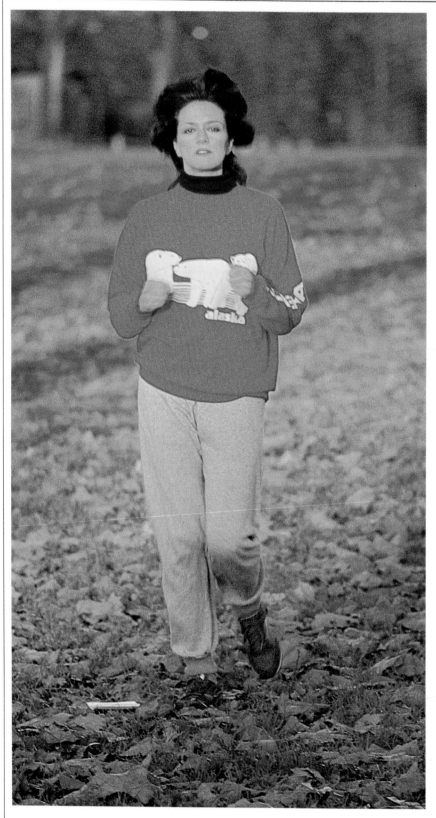

Good, well-cushioned running shoes are essential for jogging and running. You will also need shorts which allow full leg movement, a comfortable T-shirt and a well-fitting bra. A tracksuit is important for keeping warm.

The emphasis in running is on building up from approximately five minutes of jogging combined with walking on alternate days. Before beginning, it is a good idea to consult one of the books on the sport for a training schedule.

Swimming is an ideal sport for all-round fitness. It develops stamina, suppleness and strength. There is no jarring of joints (as in running) because the body is supported by water; it is therefore a good exercise for the elderly and for people with arthritis or back problems.

Cycling builds up stamina in the heart and lungs as well as increasing the strength and mobility of the legs. Like swimming, it has the advantage of not jarring the joints.

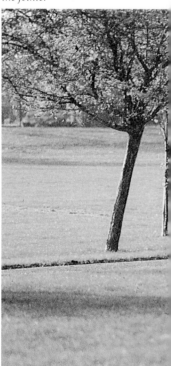

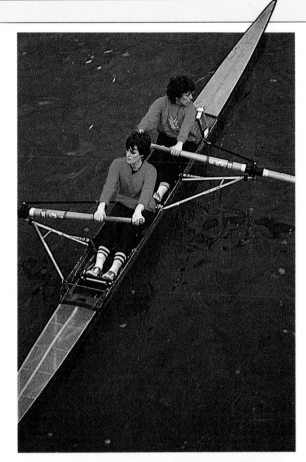

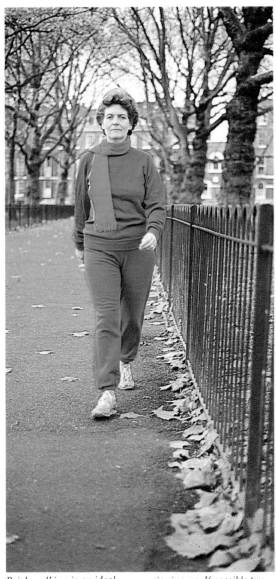

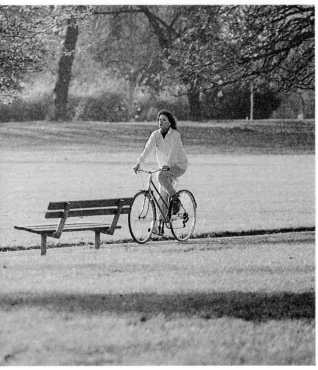

Brisk walking is an ideal form of exercise for everyone, but particularly for the elderly. If you are not tempted to venture out alone, there are many walking and rambling clubs who organize expeditions throughout the year.

Keep-fit, dance and aerobics classes are not only excellent forms of exercise but are usually very sociable, and also have the advantage of taking place in a dry, warm environment!

Look for a class with a reputable teacher, and ask to watch a session before signing up. If possible try to attend a centre which has classes at beginners, intermediate and advanced levels.

long because the muscles go into 'oxygen debt' very quickly. It is for this reason that you feel puffed when you rush up stairs or sprint. Anaerobic exercise creates a lactic acid build-up in the muscles due to the oxygen debt, and it is this that makes the muscles ache or burn. That famous rallying cry of Jane Fonda, 'Go for the burn!' thus actually encourages pupils to push their muscles beyond their capacity. Pain is a warning signal that should always be heeded; it is the body's way of telling us we need a rest.

The training effect

Yes, exercise is going to seem difficult in the beginning, but if your exercise programme is built up gradually and you have chosen something you enjoy, which gives you the determination to persist, then within a matter of weeks your capacity to intensify and prolong the activity will increase, and you will be able to do so with less fatigue.

The fundamental principle behind the training effect is that the body thrives on use. If you give your body something to do which is a little more strenuous than it has been used to, it will very soon adjust to this 'overload'. The benefits of training also come when you least expect it. When the body is at rest, strengthening and rebuilding takes place, bringing renewed vigour and a sense of refreshment.

Movement for mobility and suppleness

Although aerobic activity increases the health of your lungs and heart, making you feel more vital, it is also important to stretch fully, in a slow and deliberate way, all the muscle groups in your body. This form of exercise is the necessary complement to the more dynamic forms, and brings the benefits of joint mobility, balance, suppleness and grace. Yoga is the archetypal stretching exercise and forms the basis of all modern variations.

When you stretch, you contract and relax a muscle, squeezing out blood and cellular wastes, and allowing fresh, oxygenated blood to flow back in. This movement of blood does not depend on the heart for its circulation or on the strenuous raising of the body's metabolism. It is altogether a quieter, slower form of movement, and as such brings relaxation and a sense of calm and renewal. Your exercise programme should combine aerobic activity with some form of slower, stretching movement.

Movement for body awareness

All exercises and movement forms from the East are founded on the principles of being aware of your body, how it functions and how your energy flows. There are also a few Western forms which have these principles as their aim. The principle of 'centering' involves finding and utilizing the core of your energy flow (or chi) which comes from a place roughly in the centre of your body around the solar plexus, and is fundamental to all the martial arts. Being constantly aware of this centre, and acting from it, keeps the whole being balanced, strong and vital.

Of course, the martial arts are very much more complicated than this and in their pure form require life-long study and devotion, but for those women who are looking for a recreational form of movement that combines grace, skill and a finely-tuned awareness of their body and how it relates to its surroundings, practising an Eastern form of movement can be very satisfying.

Movement forms which are slow, flowing and emphasise awareness of the body are extremely valuable to us in the modern world of rush and hurry. For women — and for men — exercise which works in a gentle, intimate way helps us to know our bodies from the inside out and to get in touch with our inner strength, our centre and our contact with the ground. 'Grounding' is an important process; it means feeling a sense of solidity and communication with the ground — both real and metaphorical — that we stand on. We could also call it 'earthiness', and people who have that earthy quality also have a sense of self-possession which is attractive and calming. Movement for body awareness, such as T'ai Chi, yoga and contact dance, brings better posture, grounding and greater sensitivity in one's relation to self and to others.

SOME ANAEROBIC SPORTS

Circuit training involves doing a series of set exercises such as press-ups, sit-ups, star jumps, squat thrusts and so on, and repeating them for a given number of times, gradually building up the number of repetitions and circuits. Circuit training has the advantage of enabling you to do the exercises in your own home, which is particularly good in the winter when you don't feel like venturing out into rain and snow. It is best, however, to go first to a gymnasium to learn from a qualified instructor how to do these exercises properly, as you will only benefit from the correct technique.

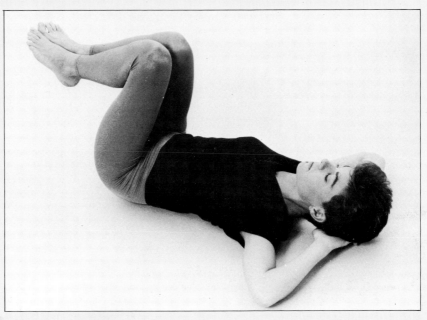

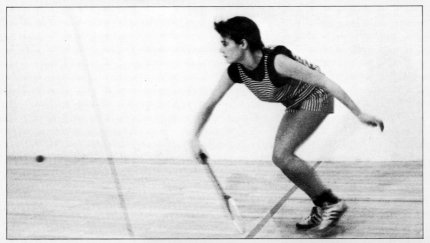

Squash and tennis are two sports which are essentially anaerobic in that the player performs in short bursts of activity, resting in between the rallies. People who love these sports swear by them, but for the beginner it is best to get fit for playing them rather than play them to get fit. Squash is far more demanding than tennis; it can be a dangerous sport to suddenly start playing especially if you are not already reasonably fit or if you have been accustomed to a sedentary lifestyle.

Weight training involves pushing and pulling a quantity of weights and repeating the lifts below your maximum ability. Smaller weights lifted many times produce stamina as well as strengthening and toning the muscles. Large loads of heavy weights lifted only a few times provide power. Many local authority run sports centres now have facilities for weight training.

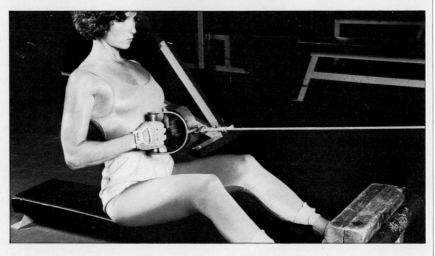

Skin and its care

Strange as it may seem, the skin is an organ. In fact, it is the largest organ of the body. It covers the entire surface, on average comprising about three square metres (20 square feet) in adults, and accounting for about one-sixth of our total body-weight.

It also varies in thickness from a mere millimetre (1/25th of an inch) on our eyelids to a comparatively thick layer of about six millimetres (a quarter of an inch) on the soles of our feet. And though subjected to continuous wear and sometimes tear, its amazing structure allows it to regenerate itself and serve us well in many important ways.

Skin consists of two main layers and a third, connecting layer.

*The outermost layer, **the epidermis**, is composed of cells with a flattened outermost surface. It contains no blood vessels, but areas subjected to heavy wear, such as the palms, contain a horny protein called keratin.*

*The under layer, **the dermis**, is considerably thicker and contains blood vessels, lymph vessels, nerves, hair follicles and about two million sweat glands.*

*The third layer, **the hypodermis**, is composed of subcutaneous tissue in which fat cells can accumulate.*

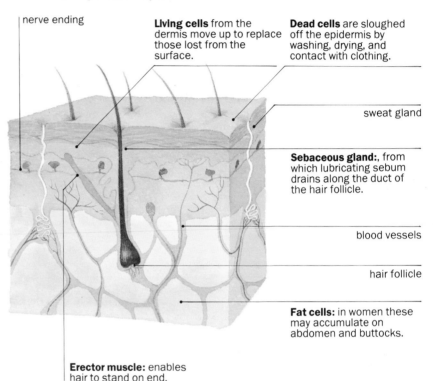

nerve ending

Living cells from the dermis move up to replace those lost from the surface.

Dead cells are sloughed off the epidermis by washing, drying, and contact with clothing.

sweat gland

Sebaceous gland:, from which lubricating sebum drains along the duct of the hair follicle.

blood vessels

hair follicle

Fat cells: in women these may accumulate on abdomen and buttocks.

Erector muscle: enables hair to stand on end.

Functions of the skin

The skin provides a perfect, protective coating — flexible enough to allow us complete freedom of movement. It is also temperature regulating, and sensitive to pain so that we have immediate warning of potential danger if we come in too close proximity with intense heat, cold or sharp objects.

Regulating temperature   Vasomotor nerves in our skin dilate or contract the blood vessels, according to the climate.
● In hot weather the blood vessels enlarge to remove heat in the form of sweat and we may lose about two litres (four pints) of fluid a day. In very hot weather it is advisable, therefore, to drink more fluids to guard against dehydration — most of us do this instinctively. (Even in temperate weather we lose about 0.5 litres (a pint) of liquid in sweat, but it evaporates as soon as it reaches the skin's surface so we are not ordinarily aware of it.) If our temperature still rises, despite the sweat loss, blood vessels in the dermis have one more trick: they dilate in order to increase the flow of warm blood to the surface of our body where it can cool down a little.
● In cold weather, the blood vessels constrict and this drives the blood inwards for a warm up. Also, our pores contract and goose pimples form, the tiny muscles of the hair follicles pull the hairs upright, and the combined force of goose pimples and hairs prevent the cold from penetrating so quickly.

Care of the skin

Apart from taking note of warning signs and acting upon them, we should pay attention to what we eat and drink and how we occupy our time as general health is reflected in the condition of the skin and our domestic and employment situations, even our pastimes affect the skin. If we have skin problems, drugs may bring temporary relief, but if we want to find a permanent cure we need to discover the underlying causes and resolve them — whether they be problems of health or stress.

Even if there is a family history of such disorders as eczema, psoriasis or acne, it does not necessarily follow that it is your genes that are to blame. It could well be that the family's lifestyle is at least partly responsible. So, eat a sensible, balanced diet; avoid stress as far as possible, get lots of fresh air, exercise — and rest — and try to keep a positive outlook on life. Worry does not do anyone any good, and it can not only harm your skin, but it can cause harm to other organs in the body.

Allergies These are well known sources of skin disorders. And in our technological society the number of possible irritants is steadily increasing: artificial fibres, soaps, washing powders and detergents, bleaches and other household chemicals, food colourants and preservatives are just a few possible irritants.

If you do suspect a particular item is creating problems, avoid it for a few days and see if the problem clears. Particularly if the suspect item is a food, you should only continue to avoid it if you do clearly benefit. If the problem

FACIAL CARE

Make-up makes you look good and feel good, but these benefits will not last unless you remove it as scrupulously as you apply it. Traces left on your skin overnight can lead to clogged pores and, eventually, to a spoiled complexion. So, however tired you are, always remove make-up last thing at night with an appropriate cleanser for your skin type: cream, milky cleansing cream or a liquid cleanser.

Eye make-up is best removed with a cleanser specifically designed for the purpose, applied on a pad of lightly moistened cotton wool or with your fingertip. Use a light touch; never scrub your skin.

If you tend to have a dry skin, after removing make-up apply a light film of moisturizer. But remember that a little goes a long way. Adding an extra amount for good measure will not be beneficial and may make your skin feel tacky!

It is a good idea to give your skin a complete rest from make-up at least once a week, but even then careful cleansing is still important, particularly if you live or work in an urban environment.

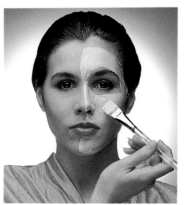

Above and right: *whatever your skin type, a mask treatment every week or so will improve circulation, cleanse and tighten pores.*

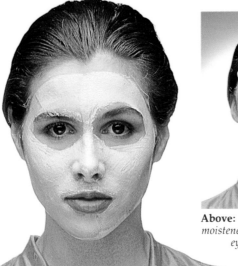

Above: *place pads of cotton wool moistened with witch hazel over your eyes, or use soothing cucumber compresses.*

persists, it may be possible for your doctor to arrange for you to have allergy tests under clinical conditions. Otherwise, you may deprive yourself of many possible 'triggers' that are not actually contributory factors at all — a miserable solution and potentially one that will do you harm rather than good.

It is sensible, however, to avoid obvious potential irritants such as harsh soaps and detergents that can alter the pH balance of your skin. If you already have an itchy skin due to using an alkaline soap, try bathing it in lukewarm water to which a dessertspoon of cider vinegar has been added — this should help to restore the correct acid content in your skin. A light moisturizing lotion or cream used after cleansing can also alleviate dryness.

Correct, deep breathing is beneficial because it tones up the other organs of elimination – the kidneys, large bowl and lungs – which, together with the skin, rid our bodies of toxins and waste matter. If skin problems do suddenly occur and you are also constipated, take the necessary corrective action because this condition can be a major contributory factor to many skin problems.

Finally, because the skin develops from the same basic cell as the nervous system, skin problems may be aggravated by nerve problems, and vice versa. Again, deep breathing can be beneficial, because it has a wonderfully calming effect on the whole body.

Hair and its care

A healthy head of hair positively glows with life — so it may come as a surprise to you to learn that it is, in fact, dead. The only part of it that is alive is the root, buried deep in a hair follicle and nourished by capillary blood vessels in the skull.

Each follicle has a long activity phase of from two to three years, during which it produces a hair that can grow to a considerable length. Then it takes a respite, the hair stops growing and, when the follicle gears up again and starts producing a new hair, the old hair is shed. That is why, no matter how gently you treat your hair, you will always find a few in your brush or comb. Only if you notice a marked increase in the amount shed, and see a visible thinning of your scalp hair, is there cause for concern, in which case you are best advised to see your doctor. Resorting to the use of commercial products without any qualified diagnosis of the cause may aggravate rather than correct the situation, and involve you in unnecesary expenditure.

Possible causes of sudden, dramatic hair loss

Any one of the following may cause many follicles to begin their rest period prematurely, causing wholesale shedding of hair, perhaps even resulting in partial, temporary baldness. Usually, replacement hair eventually grows although it may be months before the patch disappears. Try not to worry about it; you will aggravate the problem if you do. If necessary, change your hair-style instead to disguise the patch, and make sure that you eat a well-balanced diet (see pages 74-79), and get plenty of fresh air and rest – these are all positive aids to recovery.

The main cause of sudden, dramatic hair loss is very often anxiety but there may well be other reasons:
- Severe or prolonged emotional stress.
- The aftermath of a major operation.
- Heavy blood loss.
- A high temperature.
- Pregnancy.

Another cause of hair loss is any disease that affects the scalp. If this causes damage to the hair follicle, it may even result in permanent hair loss. This is another good reason why you should consult your doctor at the outset; your doctor can refer you to a dermatologist who is best qualified to attempt arrest of the disease. A trichologist (hair specialist) cannot do that.

General hair care

Hair care is not just a matter of vanity; if your hair looks good you will feel good — and anything that affects your sense of well-being is worth attention. However luxuriant your hair was as a child and teenager, if you neglect or abuse it, you will probably suffer split ends and it will be lank or brittle later in life. So have it cut or trimmed regularly, according to how quickly it grows. Wash it regularly, according to its type and where you live; if you live in the heart of a big city you almost certainly need to wash it more regularly than if you live in the country.

Nowadays you can buy shampoos for all textures and types of hair. Some make pretty extravagant claims — boasting, for instance, that they can thicken it. This is not possible, although they may leave a film on the hair shaft so that it appears thicker. It will also probably need washing more often because such a coating attracts dirt in the same way that setting lotion or lacquer can. So don't be brainwashed by the advertisers. Save your money by buying the least expensive shampoo that cleanses your hair without causing you adverse reactions.

The essential ingredient in shampoo is a detergent (which varies in concentration according to the manufacturer) to remove accumulated dust and excess grease from your hair. Most of the other ingredients, apart from something to prevent the detergent irritating your scalp, are included just to woo you: perfumes, conditioners, foam-boosters, herbs, and so on.

When you have discovered an acceptable shampoo, if you wash your hair more than once a week, one lathering should be quite sufficient. Just make sure that you dispense the shampoo evenly through your hair. Once you have worked it into a lather, leave it for just 30 seconds or so, then rinse it off thoroughly. Do not be tempted to use an extra amount for good measure — it will simply take longer to rinse.

Whether or not you need to use a conditioner depends on the health of your hair. If it is brittle from too frequent colouring or perming sessions, a

---

HAIR: COMMON COMPLAINTS

Dandruff
We all know what dandruff looks like — small particles of skin that accumulate on the scalp, then become lodged in the hair or flake off on to clothing.

Cause We shed dead skin scales all over the body every day without even noticing them, but when they accumulate on the scalp they are clearly visible. Dandruff is not infectious; it is simply the result of a cell turnover that has accelerated past the normal rate. It can occur when you are generally run down.

Treatment Do not try to remove the scales by vigorous brushing, combing or — worse — scratching with your fingernails; you might cause an

infection. If the problem is only slight, it will suffice to use a shampoo specifically designed for treatment of dandruff — one containing zinc pyrithione is most likely to help the condition.

Use it according to directions on the container. Do not use more on the principle that if a little helps then a bit extra will be better still. It won't! And don't massage your scalp vigorously when shampooing. Your scalp needs gentle treatment at such times. Keep your comb and brush scrupulously clean.

A simple, herbal treatment for dandruff consists of boiling four tablespoons of dried thyme in two cups of water for ten minutes. Strain the mixture and cool. After shampooing pour one cup over your damp

hair and massage gently. Do not rinse off, but dry your hair as normal. This makes enough for two treatments.

Ringworm (tinea)
This fungal infection of the scalp is identifiable by irritation and circular, pink, scaly patches on the skin. They may sometimes weep. This is a contagious disease.

Treatment This is not a complaint that you can treat efficiently yourself. Go to your doctor, who can prescribe an anti-fungal cream not available over the counter. And do not wait to see if it will clear up of its own accord. The sooner treatment begins, the easier it is to eradicate.

conditioner may help. But the sensible thing is to give your hair a few months to recover before subjecting it to further treatments of that kind. Perms and dyes are usually strongly alkaline, and therefore disturb the hair's natural pH balance. And because they distort the keratin scales, the hair tends to become wiry and difficult to comb through.

Some dos and don'ts for hair care

- Do use a wide-toothed comb to untangle wet or damp hair. A fine one will drag on the hair and may even tug it out.
- Do hold each section of the hair as you comb it through and gently comb the length below your hand, ie furthest away from your scalp. This safeguards against tugging the hair out by the roots if you encounter a particularly stubborn tangle.
- Do towel-dry your hair at least every other time you wash it, to protect it from the drying effects of electric blow-dryers, or electric rollers.
- Do, if you must use heated rollers, first wind a tissue around the ends of your hair to protect it a little.
- Don't colour-shampoo your hair a second or third time in rapid succession after a first result that was a disappointment.
- Don't do a full-head home perm until you have done a test curl as instructed, even if you have used that particular brand successfully before. You may in the meantime have developed an allergy and so create terrible problems for yourself.
- Don't use spiky brush rollers; remove the inner brush and use the roller on its own. Better still, use cushioned rollers or strips of twisted rag instead.
- Don't sunbathe after perming or tinting your hair, unless you wear some head protection — a sun hat or scarf. Without it you risk having very dry, brittle hair.

Eyes and their care

If you have ever had an eye infection or an injury that has necessitated wearing an eye-patch for a brief period, you will appreciate the importance and desirability of having both eyes in good working order, to maintain a balanced perspective of the world around you. To help you to treat your eyes with due respect, here is basic information on the structure of the eyes, how they work and how best to care for them.

Eye care

If you have normal vision, your eyes will ordinarily take care of themselves — thanks to the tear-washing process described above. But if you begin to have any of the following problems, it is sensible to visit your doctor for advice without delay.
- Deterioration of vision, involving a generalized blur or a centralized blur, loss of side vision, double vision, flashing lights and spots before your eyes, or general eye strain.
- Swollen lids or reddened white of the eye.
- Discharge.
- Pain.

Your doctor will either prescribe treatment (possibly drops or ointment), refer you to an optician or, if he detects a more serious condition, refer you to an ophthalmologist (a medically qualified doctor with specialist interest in the eyes). To check initially, your doctor may:
- Test the eye muscles to detect a squint or any tendency to squint.
- Examine the lids for styes, the whites of the eyes for conjunctivitis, and the cornea for abrasions.

Examination of the eyes can also reveal whether you have:
- Cataracts.
- Glaucoma.
- An illness such as diabetes.

HOW THE EYE WORKS

The structure of the eye: *each eye is spheroid and about 2.5cm (1in) in diameter. The eyelid covers about two-thirds of the front of each eyeball and, at the inner corner, each eye has a small, fleshy pad.*

A tear gland in the upper lid produces a film of tears with every blink to clean and sterilize the eye. The 'tears' then drain away through tear ducts, into the back of the nose.

The diagram shows the main structures of the eye.

Sclera: protective tissue.

Choroid: a pigmented membrane.

Cornea: window of the eye — lets in light.

Pupil: 'black hole' — light passes through.

Lens: focuses received light on to retina.

Aqueous humour: nourishes the lens.

Iris: regulates light through cornea.

Vitreous humour: preserves shape of eyeball.

Retina: receives image from lens.

Optic nerve: transmits 'coded' image to brain.

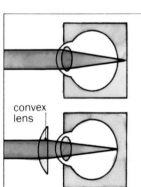

Far-sightedness *(or hypermetropia) occurs because the eyeball is slightly more curved than is 'normal', thus causing the lens to focus behind the retina. Only distant objects can be seen clearly. The problem can be corrected by using spectacles with convex-shaped lenses.*

convex lens

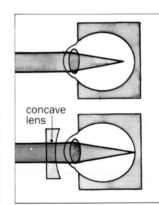

Near-sightedness *(or myopia) occurs when the eyeball is slightly less curved than 'normal'. In this case, the lens of the eye will focus in front of the retina, blurring all objects except those close by. The refractive error can be corrected by spectacles with concave lenses.*

concave lens

The eye is like a camera, with the lens sited towards the front of the eye and held in position by the ciliary muscle, which helps it to focus near or distant objects. Light enters the eye through the cornea and is then controlled by the iris, where tiny muscles constrict or dilate the size of the pupil — the 'black hole' through which the light reaches the lens.

In turn, the lens focuses the light on to the retina lying at the back of the eye. The retina transforms the light into coded impulses, passed on to the brain via the optic nerve.

The brain then decodes the impulses in such a way that you see things the right way up and the right way round. (They reach the back of the brain transposed left to right — and upside down.)

Going to an optician

An optician tests your eyes for focusing errors, for which he or she can then prescribe glasses and/or contact lenses. An optician is also trained to recognize eye diseases but cannot treat them. If he or she suspects an eye complaint you will be referred to an eye specialist — an opthalmologist — who will repeat the same tests but in even greater detail, and will also carry out other more specific tests.

Testing for distance vision

Each eye is covered in turn while you read letters of gradually decreasing size on a wall-chart at a distance of 6m (18ft) from you, to see how many lines you can read without strain.

Testing for near vision

You will be asked to read from print in various type-sizes, held at a normal reading distance from you.

Don't be nervous if an adjustable light or pen torch is shone into your eyes. It is rather disturbing if you are already in an anxious state, but no pain is involved and you can console yourself with the thought that if something is wrong, such a thorough search will detect it so that it can be treated before it worsens. If your doctor detects a medical problem he or she will decide on the correct course of action; if the problem is one of long or short sight you will then be advised to visit an optician.

Preventing eye injury

Many eye injuries could be avoided if only sensible precautions were taken when participating in certain sports, engaging in certain types of work, or carrying out DIY tasks around the home. It is always sensible to wear protective goggles:
● When using chemicals, painting or spraying with creosote, hammering, drilling, sawing or sanding or hedge-clipping with a power-driven cutter.
● When engaged in sports during which you may be hit in the face — squash, cricket, badminton, and fencing in particular.
● When protective goggles are standard issue in your line of work. They would not be provided if there was no likely danger. Furthermore, if you do not wear them and then suffer injury, you are unlikely to receive any compensation.

Emergency eye treatment

Removing a foreign body from the eye First try blinking rapidly once or twice to encourage an increased tear-flow, which may well dislodge the foreign body. If not, gently grasp the eyelashes of the upper lid between thumb and forefinger and pull the upper lid down over the lower one; hold for a few seconds, then release.

If this fails, waste no more time. Put a protective pad over the eye and go to see your doctor without further delay. Do not rub the eye if you can possibly resist; you will simply aggravate the problem and possibly scratch the conjunctiva.

Treatment for accidents with chemicals

Bathe the eye immediately under fresh, cold, running water. Take care to tilt your head so that water trickling from the damaged eye cannot enter the other one and cause further problems. Hold your eyelids open with one hand so that the water can really do its work. Keep up the bathing treatment for at least 10 minutes, even if the burning sensation eases. Then cover the eye with a sterile pad and go to see your doctor, even if you feel better.

Sight is a precious gift and it is sensible, therefore, to always check up on any problem with your doctor. For this reason no specific information about treating general eye problems is given here, other than suggestions on dealing with emergency situations.

Ears and their care

A normal human being starts life with acutely keen hearing — a sensory gift to be treasured because, without it, our technological society would be highly dangerous to live in. We would not hear the warning roar of approaching fast traffic, or a cry of 'look out' if we needed to move quickly in order to avoid being hit by some falling object. And we would have none of the pleasures of listening to music, or to the talk of family, friends and colleagues. After a time, the lack of such audio experiences might even cause us to speak less intelligibly, because we would not be able to hear the sounds we were making. In fact, children who are born deaf have considerable difficulty in learning to speak, and special tuition is necessary.

So, how do we hear, and how can we protect this ability? In this respect, it may be helpful, first, to look at the illustration (right) which shows how the ears are structured and how they function, because this is essential to any real understanding of why and how hearing problems can arise.

Structure of the ear: the external ear *consists of the ear flap (pinna), and a curvy, tubular, skin-lined passage (the external canal) that passes on collected sound via the eardrum (tympanic membrane) which vibrates as sound reaches it.*
The middle ear *(tympanic cavity) is a small bony cavity containing air and three tiny bones (ossicles) suspended across it which transmit the vibrations picked up from the eardrum to the:*
Inner ear *is a labyrinth of tubes containing the sense receptors: the cochlea for hearing; the vestibule to keep us right way up, and the three semi-circular canals that enable us to maintain our balance.*

External canal: conveys sound vibrations to the eardrum.

Semicircular canals: enable us to maintain our sense of balance.

Vestibule: keeps us aware of the pull of gravity, so that we remain the right way up.

Cochlea:, the sense receptor enabling us to hear.

Eardrum (tympanic membrane): connects the external and middle ear, and passes on the vibrations.

Pinna and lobe: collect the sound waves.

Ossicles (the malleus, incus and stapes): transmits the vibrations to the inner ear.

The process of hearing

Our hearing is so sensitive that we can distinguish about 370 changes in volume level, and a staggering 2,000 variations in pitch.
• Our reception of the volume of sound depends on the amplitude of the sound wave — the greater the amplitude, the louder the sound we hear.
• Our reception of pitch is governed by the frequency of the sound — the higher the frequency, the higher the pitch we hear.
We can also distinguish the direction from which any sound originates:
• If the sound occurs directly behind, or directly in front of us, both ears will receive it in equal volume and the brain will interpret the signals to locate the source of sound accordingly.
• If the sound comes from one side of us, one ear will receive it more loudly and, again, the brain will interpret the signals, and, noting the difference in volume between them, will pinpoint the source of the sound.

Care of the ears

Keep the outer ear clean, of course, but never try to remove wax with a cotton bud, or prod your ear with any similar object. The eardrum is highly sensitive and you may push hardened wax even further into the ear canal, or do yourself other, permanent damage.
If you have any ear problem, go to see your doctor and get a proper diagnosis. If it is simply accumulated wax, drops can be prescribed to soften the wax and, after the drops have been used for a few days, the ears can be syringed by the doctor or an assistant. If the problem is more serious, treatment can begin without delay.
• If you are provided with ear muffs because you are engaged in particularly noisy work, be sensible and wear them.
• If you frequently listen to music and wear earphones for this purpose, keep the volume reasonably low. And if you use earplugs, keep them scrupulously clean to avoid possibility of an ear infection.
• If you have any infection of the teeth or throat, don't neglect it; otherwise it may spread to your ears.

COMMON EAR PROBLEMS AND THEIR TREATMENT

Mastoiditis This occurs when a middle-ear infection spreads to the mastoid bone, behind the ear. The bone swells, causing pain and fever.

If the condition is not too serious, it may respond to antibiotics. Otherwise, surgical removal of the infected bone may be necessary.

Menière's Disease This is a disorder of the labryinth in the inner ear, and can seriously affect one's sense of balance, causing sudden attacks of vertigo. These attacks may be accompanied by tinnitus and rapid, uneven movements of the eyeball, which have the disturbing effect of making stationary objects appear to whirl around. There may also be nausea and vomiting.

Attacks may last for several days and, like migraine, may recur within days or weeks; similarly they may not recur for months.

Recovery is often spontaneous, but if the attack causes severe discomfort, anti-nausea drugs, sedatives or diuretics may be prescribed.

Otitis media This is a middle-ear infection in which the eardrum becomes swollen and red, and may perforate. There may be temporary deafness, ringing in the ear, pain and fever.

If this condition is not treated quickly, permanent deafness may result. Fortunately, with timely treatment, the inflammation can be successfully dealt with

and hearing restored. So, if you have the symptoms described, do see your doctor without delay.

Tinnitus (ringing in the ears) This is often accompanied by dizzy spells or loss of balance. Tinnitus can be caused by high blood pressure, particularly if you are taking certain antibiotics or aspirin; but do not stop taking them. Instead, go to see your doctor so that a preliminary investigation can be made and, if necessary, you can be referred for specialist treatment. These symptoms may also be experienced with certain ear diseases.

Hearing problems

There are two main forms of deafness: the first is caused by a physical problem such as inflammation of the eardrum; the second results from damage to the nerves of the ear.

Conductive deafness is when the transmission of sound waves is affected by an abscess or inflammation of the eardrum; by a physical blockage such as can be formed by accumulated wax; or adhesion of the tiny ear bones in the middle ear, or gradual thickening of the oval window leading to the inner ear. In this form of deafness, a hearing aid can be helpful.

Perceptive or nerve deafness is when damage to nerve pathways or sensory cells is the cause of hearing loss. In such cases, a hearing aid is of little use.

To assess which kind of deafness has occurred, a tuning fork is used. If the vibrating fork is held just a short distance from the ear, the sound waves emitted will have to be transmitted through the middle ear in order to be heard. If, however, the middle ear is blocked or diseased, the sound will be heard indistinctly, if at all.

Then the vibrating fork will be held to the skull because, if the cochlea is healthy, it can pick up the sound waves emitted at that point without them first having to pass through the middle ear. If, however, the cochlea or auditory nerve is diseased, the conduction of sound will be lessened or non-existent. This is perceptive hearing loss.

● **Babies** may be born deaf due to an underdeveloped internal ear, or damage incurred in the early, formative weeks of pregnancy.

● **In childhood**, the most common causes of deafness (perceptive hearing loss) are meningitis or chronic infection spreading from the middle ear.

● **In adults**, particularly in women, the most common cause is hereditary otosclerosis — hardening of the tissues in the middle ear. Surgery may bring about some improvement in hearing, but the process cannot usually be halted.

Teeth and their care

Regular cleaning is essential for healthy teeth. Otherwise, carbohydrates in the food you eat will be transformed into acid by bacteria naturally present in your mouth. The acid gradually breaks down the protective enamel and, once it has invaded the dentine, quickly creates a cavity. Toothache will follow and, if you don't seek dental treatment quickly, you could have an abscess, too. Quite apart from suffering pain and a swollen face, both of which could have been prevented, you may lose the tooth if neglect has continued to the point where draining the abscess and treatment with antibiotics cannot help.

Care of the gums is as important as care of the teeth. If less than thorough, brushing leaves food fragments lodged between your teeth, a deposit called plaque may form and work its way down the sides of the tooth, gradually attacking the supportive gum and creating 'pockets' into which more bacteria can find their way. As a result you will have very sore gums and, eventually, loose teeth. A great many otherwise healthy teeth are lost in this way .

Fortunately, you can prevent such calamities by scrupulously cleaning your teeth and gums after meals or, at least, after breakfast each morning and again last thing at night. Follow the routine illustrated below and you should have no problems.

Caring for your teeth

HOW TO CLEAN YOUR TEETH

Use a brush with a small to medium-sized head, and close-set, straight-topped bristles. Replace the brush as soon as it shows signs of splaying. If it splays out in under three months, try a different brand of brush. If the same thing happens you may be scrubbing rather than brushing your teeth — with consequent wear on the enamel.

Use dental sticks and/or dental floss to remove any food still lodged between your teeth after brushing them. Waxed floss tends to be easier to use than the unwaxed variety. There's even a floss now with a 'threader' end so you can easily insert it between your teeth at gum level if they are too close to slide floss up between them.

Once a week check up on how efficiently you have been cleaning your teeth by using a disclosing tablet that leaves tell-tale colour on the tooth surface wherever plaque is beginning to form. Having been thus warned, simply brush your teeth again until all the colour has been removed.

Whichever type of toothpaste you use, be sparing with it; otherwise the speedy lather will cause you to spit out and rinse before you've really brushed them efficiently.

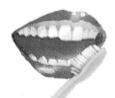

On your upper teeth, brush downwards, taking care to include the gum area. Then repeat the action, only this time brushing upwards, to clean your lower teeth.

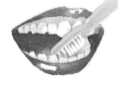

Brush the backs of both upper and lower teeth just as thoroughly, tilting the brush to the angle shown, as necessary, to ensure that you also brush in between each tooth at gum level where food particles can lodge if you are not scrupulous enough.

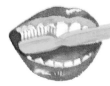

Brush the cutting or grinding edge of your teeth, using a rotating action to get into every tiny crevice.

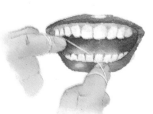

Finally, wind a length of dental floss around your fingers, as shown, and use it to remove any remaining debris.

Emotional and mental well-being

**The psychological
approach**

Because of the complicated situation that now exists in modern psychology, people have become uncertain as to exactly what the different branches of the profession do, when they come into action, and whether they provide a form of medicine for the sick, a popular therapeutic pastime for wealthy neurotics or a path to personal growth and self awareness that anyone may choose to follow. Some definitions:

Psychology is the science of the nature, functions and phenomena of the human mind. Therefore a psychologist may have nothing to do with the medical profession but may be a teacher or student of the science. Clinical psychologists have a degree in psychology and sometimes sociology as well, and have then undergone further training in counselling skills. This has become a recognized profession.

Psychiatry is the medical treatment of 'diseases of the mind', and all psychiatrists undergo medical training. As doctors, however, their training gives them a tendency to rely heavily on drugs and (though increasingly less) on medical technology such as electro-convulsive therapy (ECT).

Psychoanalysis began with Freud, who analyzed the origins of pathological, mental or nervous disorders through talking to his patients and exploring with them their past, their relationships, their likes and dislikes, their avoidances and obsessions, as a means of treating the deep causes of their disorders. Psychoanalysis has developed a great deal since Freud through the work of such eminent figures as Jung, Adler and others, although traditional psychoanalysis is practised today in much the same way as in Freud's time, mostly in the private sector. It can be a costly and lengthy business involving hourly sessions two, three or even five times a week, sometimes for several years. All psychoanalysts have to go through lengthy analysis themselves and be trained at one of the recognized institutes in this country before they can set up a practice.

Psychotherapy is a much broader term and includes any therapy of a psychological nature. It is often used in referring to the newer humanistic psychotherapies which developed from the 1930s onwards out of a sense of the limitations of traditional psychoanalysis in the Freudian or Jungian mould. The essential difference between analysis and psychotherapy is that the latter approaches each patient as an individual rather than on the basis of a set methodology. Psychotherapy encompasses a wide range of diverse techniques including counselling, bioenergetics, Rogerian therapy, *Gestalt*, psychodrama, group work and self-discovery through painting and writing. On a one-to-one basis a session is directed by the client according to his or her wishes and needs, and to the particular training of the therapist. The length of time a person may see a therapist can vary from a couple of diagnostic meetings to a weekly session for several years. This will depend on the individual.

A group workshop may be determined by a theme or common aim, at which the therapist may act as a facilitator or direct the group's use of the time available. In fact the 'growth group' is a common feature of the approach of psychotherapy. Individuals meet, usually weekly, and explore together personal issues, usually with a therapist to act as guide.

The emphasis in psychotherapy is less on a relationship between the healer and the patient, more about individuals engaged in helping the client gain insight into his or her problems through self-awareness.

SLEEPING PILLS AND TRANQUILLIZERS

Every woman who is offered a prescription should ask what are the actions and possible side effects of the drug being prescribed. If it is explained to you that these are tranquillizers and will make you feel calmer, you need to consider whether you really would feel better if you suffered any of the common side effects of the drugs. In the *British National Formulary*, the annual authoritative publication on drugs and their uses, the possible side effects of Valium (the most commonly prescribed tranquillizer) are listed as drowsiness, dizziness, unsteadiness, confusion, dry mouth, and hypersensitivity reactions, including skin rashes and breathing difficulties.

In terms of the ultimate benefits of these drugs, you alone must decide whether their sedative effects are worth risking any or all of these side effects. The *British National Formulary* does not provide much information regarding long-term addiction but it states quite clearly: 'Although there is a tendency to prescribe these drugs to almost anyone with stress-related symptoms, unhappiness, or minor physical disease, their use in many situations is unjustified.'

Long-term dependency on sleeping pills and tranquillizers is common. The most serious long-term effect is that it has a depressant, and sometimes paralysing, action on our decision-making ability.

All drugs and so-called stimulants, like alcohol, cigarettes and coffee, ultimately have a depressant effect on the body (and on the mind) by slowing down the conduction of nerve stimuli in the brain and supressing the action of the hypothalamus (our alarm apparatus). The hypothalamus initiates our reactions to fear, sex and sleep, so suppression of its activity can result in disturbed behaviour in all of these areas. Dreaming sleep is suppressed by sleeping pills, and some of the most unpleasant withdrawal symptoms after stopping the pills are nightmares, interrupted sleep, and frightening fantasies as the body over-compensates and re-adjusts after such deprivation. Other withdrawal symptoms include shivering, shaking, suicidal depression, extreme fatigue, severe anxiety and confusion.

- 34 per cent of British women have been prescribed tranquillizers or sleeping pills at some time.
- 75 per cent of the 13 million prescriptions written annually for tranquillizers are for women. This means that every year, nearly 10 million women take tranquillizers.
- Tranquillizers work by damping down intelligence and self-perception.

Today, many different agencies and individuals practise psychotherapeutic techniques, from the doctor who behaves in a caring way towards his patients, helping them through crises in their lives, to social workers, marriage-guidance counsellors, clinical theologians and trained psychologists.

How to find a psychotherapist Some general practices include either a clinical psychologist or a psychotherapist, or both, but most do not. If you decide you need counselling or psychotherapy, discuss this with your doctor. If no advice or help is forthcoming, you should then decide whether you need individual psychotherapy or group psychotherapy, or whether to join one of the many self-help groups instead. There are self-help groups for practically every problem, from those suffering from muscular dystrophy to compulsive eating. Many psychotherapists also practice group work or are able to put you in touch with someone who does.

It is far better, in almost all cases, to try the human approach rather than to take drugs, whether they are prescribed by your doctor or by a psychiatrist. In many ways the psychotherapist today fills a role that used to be filled by a close friend, a relative or the parish priest. Some women actually prefer to confide in someone outside their close circle. They feel they can no longer go on burdening friends.

As is evident in the next section on stress, many of our problems are self-generated and more to do with our perception of pressures than with the actual pressures themselves. There are simple self-help techniques to deal with stress and to help you avoid the breakdown of your coping mechanisms.

Coping with stress

Our modern world presents all women with more challenges, demands, opportunities and choices than we have ever had before. Life moves faster than it did, with a multiplicity of claims on our time, attention, involvement, commitment and energy. Our choice of work is greater, with positions of responsibility and creativity open to us where once they were not. We are offered a wider range of stimuli to attract and distract us: films, television, videos, books, and a range of activities from women's groups and politics to evening classes in car maintenance or flower arranging. We rarely rest, there is always so much to do . . . to the point where we find it hard to know where to turn. Add to this the invasion even of the home — a woman's traditional nest and retreat — by the telephone and the demands of young children, and we can see that the fabled peace of the household (if it ever truly existed) is certainly something of a myth. Home may be neither a place of respite and recuperation for a woman after work, nor a guarantee of an unstressful life for women who are there all day.

Our lives have become so full of noise and activity that we have lost sight of the need for silence and stillness, the vital balance for fulfilled life. The lack of this balance can so easily turn what should be exciting challenges and possibilities into sources of stress. Each of us responds differently; we may feel overwhelmed, exhausted, depressed and weary. We become ill or irritable, feel angry, trapped, frightened, anxious or permanently tense. Our bodies, too, respond with backaches and muscle tension in the neck, stomach, throat and elsewhere. We become emotional in inappropriate situations or snap at loved ones, over-react to demands at home and at work.

Women are particularly vulnerable to stress today because, for the first time we are not bound by tradition; we are making choices as to how we want to live our lives and having to balance several roles. It is not so much the choice in itself which is stressful, but rather that we are being expected, and expect ourselves, to make intelligent, positive and appropriate decisions which will radically and permanently affect the shape of our lives, without having been taught how to choose. We have had our expectations raised by the women's movement, the press and media — and these do not always coincide with the reality of our capacities and our situation.

Making sensible, constructive choices involves balancing pros and cons, facing reality rather than how one would wish things to be, assessing a number of factors from finances to personality and close relationships. It also involves taking risks, having the courage to go with a vision or an ideal rather than being side-tracked by 'advice', by comparing ourselves to others, by social conventions or stereotypes. All this is a skill, and a difficult one, which must be learnt. Women have had only a few decades to pick up the skill of life-management and yet we find ourselves having to cope in a social world still in a state of transition which demands clear-sightedness from all of us.

All this sets up a lot of stress, confusion, and feelings of inadequacy and anxiety — concern, for instance, that if we choose to work our children will suffer, or that if we choose to stay at home people will think we are 'just a housewife'. Research studies confirm that women are liable to suffer more stress today for all these reasons.

The importance of relaxation

One solution to stress is to change our living circumstances. For instance, if we have always been city-dwellers, we may find it possible to move to the country, away from the tensions of city life. Or we may alter our responses to the sources of stress. The first solution, even if it were desirable or possible for most people, is a false one. The very business of living, whether in the country or the city, involves us in unavoidable stressful situations from births, relationships, illness and death to examinations, board meetings, rush-hour travel, work deadlines, coping with small children, and so on.

Some fortunate people have such a sanguine temperament that they can emerge unflustered from even the most stressful situations. They can make their daily journey to work during the rush hour reading a book or just pondering inner thoughts, remaining calm and conserving their energy for the day ahead. For many others, the journey itself causes tension and irritation. They are frustrated by the delays, and become claustrophobic on crowded buses, trains or tubes, feeling threatened by the pressure of so many bodies. Blood pressure rises, adrenalin and noradrenaline are secreted into the blood stream, muscles tense, teeth are clenched, heads throb and bodies are keyed up and exhausted before the working day begins. Most of us have, at times, experienced this or similar situations.

Although relaxation techniques cannot magically transform us into calm human beings who remain impervious to stress, if practised regularly they can help us to cultivate a greater awareness of self, a greater sensitivity to the way our bodies function, and to control and quieten the stress responses.

It is important, however, that anyone practising a relaxation technique should do so regularly, preferably every day, because in this way it becomes absorbed into the pattern of life. You don't have to think about it, or make a conscious effort to fit it in. Otherwise, it would be so easy for this discipline to become simply another source of stress.

The second reason for practising relaxation techniques regularly is that the effects are cumulative. Like any retraining of the body, and particularly one that involves the weaning of the body away from an addiction (whether cigarettes, alcohol or stress), it takes time.

Also, you should practise relaxation techniques without expectations. Make this one area of your life which is *not* goal-oriented, where you do *not* have to achieve anything, compete with anyone or please anyone but yourself. This is your time, your space, in which to get to know yourself and your inner centre. The techniques help you to release consciously your whole body, and involve getting to know where and how to hold tension and how to release that tension. They focus in turn on different parts of the body — limbs, stomach, neck, head — allowing you to relax each until your whole body is still, relaxed and peaceful. This state is quite different from that of 'flopping'. You feel very alert and aware, without being tense.

Gradually you can incorporate what you learn into your daily life even when not consciously practising the technique. You become tuned to recognizing points and moments of tension and are able to release and let go of these causes of stress without going through the full relaxation process.

Sleep patterns

Remember that no amount of practising a technique can supplant good, deep sleep. Sleep is a healer, and we all need it to regenerate our bodies, to repair and restore tissues, cells and the immune system. The quality of our sleep is important too. If we sleep lightly or curled up in tension we are unlikely to awaken refreshed. We have already seen that dreaming is also a vital part of sleep — each night we move several times between 'orthodox' or dreamless sleep and the dreaming state called REM. Sleeping pills inhibit REM sleep and, if deprived of this regularly, we become irritable, restless or anxious. Regular practise of a relaxation technique can improve the quality of your sleep.

SLEEP AND RELAXATION

A state somewhere between waking and dreaming characterizes the first period of sleep. Gradually there is a falling off in muscular tension and the body functions slow right down until the deepest stage of sleep is reached — a stage termed NREM sleep, which stands for non-rapid eye movement.

NREM sleep is followed by a lighter, dreaming phase in which the closed eyes move rapidly — hence the name REM sleep. During these phases the electrical brain waves speed up; heart rate, breathing and blood pressure undergo rapid fluctuations, especially during a flurry of rapid eye movement. Most of the body's muscles are relaxed, although in men the penis may be erect. Blood flows rapidly through the brain; its constituent cells

are being renewed.

In the NREM phases, brain waves are large and slow and the growth hormone is pumped into the blood to repair and renew skin and other tissues.

The whole cycle, from dropping off to sleep to the end of the first dreaming phase (REM sleep) takes less than two hours.

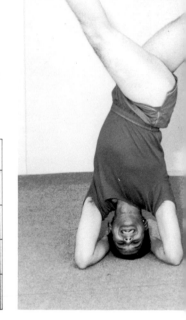

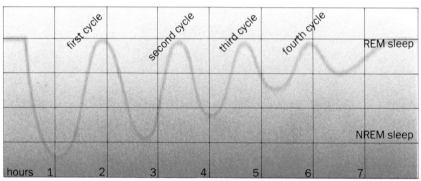

Yoga

Beginners must be taught Hatha Yoga by a competent teacher. It is a practical exercise system designed to work with and through the body to expand awareness. The postures (asanas) are practised slowly and rhythmically, and affect the central nervous system and the glandular, structural and organic systems of the body.

Yoga means union or integration, and this is the effect it has on those who practise the combination of physical stretching and twisting, the controlled and conscious breathing which accompanies every posture, and the concentration brought to bear on the movement. It is also a very good complement to strenuous physical activity, focusing as it does on calm, concentrated sustained stretch. When you have mastered the principles and postures you can practise yoga alone at home, although it is also a continuous learning process and most people prefer to attend a regular weekly class.

Complete relaxation

Complete relaxation involves focusing your mind on each part of your body in turn until the whole of you is completely relaxed. The process takes about 15 minutes and is performed lying down with closed eyes and with your arms by your sides. You may find it comfortable to have a small cushion under your knees. Focus your total attention on each section of your body in turn, starting with your feet, and gently repeat to yourself inwardly a few times, 'My feet are completely relaxed.' See in your mind's eye and feel your feet become deeply relaxed. Progress to relax each part of your body in turn, from ankles to calves, thighs, stomach, hips, back, neck, right up to the top of your head; then relax your shoulders, arms and hands, until completely relaxed.

Lie quietly, feeling the weight of your muscles supported by the floor or bed. If you want to sink even deeper into a relaxed state you have only to tell yourself, 'I am getting more and more relaxed, sinking deeper and deeper.' This form of self-hypnosis is very effective. You should feel the slight warm tingling of the blood and energy now going freely up and down your body and

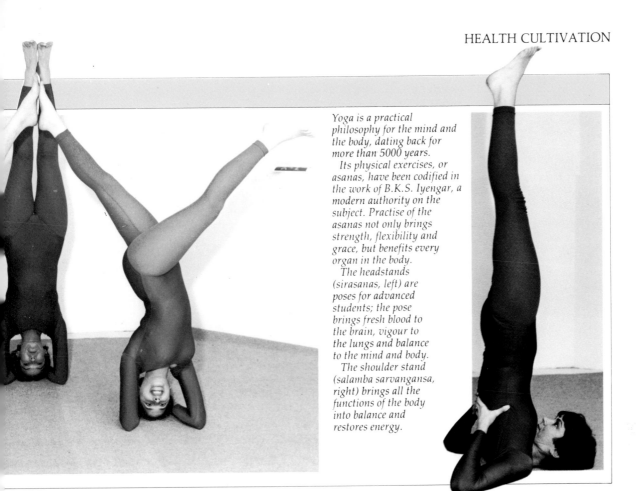

Yoga is a practical philosophy for the mind and the body, dating back for more than 5000 years.

Its physical exercises, or asanas, have been codified in the work of B.K.S. Iyengar, a modern authority on the subject. Practise of the asanas not only brings strength, flexibility and grace, but benefits every organ in the body.

The headstands (sirasanas, left) are poses for advanced students; the pose brings fresh blood to the brain, vigour to the lungs and balance to the mind and body.

The shoulder stand (salamba sarvangansa, right) brings all the functions of the body into balance and restores energy.

your mind should be still but open and aware. Afterwards you will feel refreshed and at peace with yourself.

Stretch relaxation

Another way to relax parts of your body is to tense and stretch them fully first. You can do this for your whole body, focusing on each part for a few seconds for a 15-minute sequence as in the previous technique, or you can spend a few minutes at your desk or in the middle of the day just tensing and relaxing specific areas prone to tension, such as the neck and shoulder region, or thighs and abdominal area. The tensing is done with an inhalation, and the relaxation with an exhalation. Keep all movements steady and rhythmic

Massage

Massage is a marvellous way to relax tight muscles. Many of us still think of massage in the Swedish massage image: a whole body massage, vigorous or even painful, lengthy and expensive. However, there are many gentler forms and also areas you can massage for yourself.

Swedish massage Uses stroking, kneading, pressure and percussion movements for both remedial and general health massage. It is called 'Swedish massage' because it was developed by Peter Henri Ling, the Swedish gymnast who established the renowned massage school in Stockholm.

Shiatsu Sometimes called acupressure, uses the fingers (shi) to apply pressure (atsu) to particular points on the body associated with the vital organs, to release and stimulate energy flow.

Intuitive massage This involves using a variety of techniques, according to what the practitioner feels to be appropriate for the individual and what the client desires: stroking, kneading, friction, holding, pulsing or pressure. The principles are to remain constantly in hand contact with the body you are massaging and allow your sense of the person's body and her voiced guidance to direct your movements. This is a gentle form of massage, relying mainly on light and heavy stroking movements.

Whereas the first two forms of massage need to be practised by a trained therapist, anyone can learn the basics of intuitive massage. A general principle is to massage towards the heart and not to massage varicose veins or areas of skin infection.

Alexander Technique

The principle of this technique, devised by F.M. Alexander in the late nineteenth and early twentieth centuries, is that of unlearning bad habits and the unhealthy ways we use our bodies (in sitting, standing, walking and so on) and replacing them with better ways of functioning. An Australian who worked as an actor, Alexander's career came to an end when he lost his voice on stage. He found that the cause of this problem was his tendency to pull his head back, shortening the back of his neck. By lifting his head and lengthening his spine, he found that correct posture could solve the problem.

Practice of the Alexander Technique has a beneficial effect on body tension and our ability to cope with stress, and it has another benefit for women. Forty per cent of women consult a doctor for back pain during their lives, and although the Alexander Technique may not necessarily provide immediate relief, as a long-term learning process it can be invaluable in freeing us from recurrence of these pains, as well as enhancing our health and energy generally, because it focuses on the spine and posture.

The Feldenkrais Method

Whereas the Alexander Technique tends to focus on the spine and on posture, another body re-education method, the Feldenkrais Method focuses on the neuro-muscular patterns in the body. Developed over many years since the 1940s by Moshe Feldenkrais, ex-sportsman and judo black belt, this method is well known in the United States and is rapidly gaining recognition over here.

One of the beauties of Feldenkrais exercises is that they are done lying down, which both reduces the gravitational pull on the spine and induces a more relaxed attitude in the student. Group classes are called Awareness Through Movement and follow a set pattern of gentle, repetitive exercises designed to increase awareness of the functioning of the various parts of the body. Private lessons, called Functional Integration, follow the needs of the individual and are generally given for remedial purposes.

Both the Alexander Technique and the Feldenkrais Method have in common the principle that the body reflects the mind, and vice versa. Our bad postural and functioning habits are as individual to us as our personality traits, and reflect similar sloppy or distorted patterns of thought. The other principle central to both techniques is the conviction that through the body we can affect and change our minds and our feelings. Depression may thus show up in a depressed, slouching or held-in body posture. Through retraining the body the emotional pattern can also be unlearned; both can be replaced with a well-tuned, better functioning mind/body whole.

Breathing techniques

There are a number of breathing exercises which you can practise for yourself and which are helpful in relaxing your whole body. When we are emotionally distressed we breathe fast or arhythmically, or hold our breath for a few seconds between inhalation and exhalation, and when we are tense we inhibit our breathing. In fact many people only breathe with about a quarter of their lung capacity a great deal of the time. The rhythm of the lungs and the ability to take in oxygen and metabolize it are closely connected with neurological functioning, so becoming aware of and enhancing your breathing should have a beneficial effect on your nerves and state of mind.

Diaphragmatic breathing   This is deep breathing. Lie on your back with one hand on your abdomen and the other on your chest. Concentrate on filling the lower part of your lungs with a slow, deep breath, then exhale slowly. The hand on your abdomen should rise as you inhale and sink as you exhale. The hand on your chest should hardly move at all. Do this exercise for 10 to 15 minutes before you go to sleep.

Even breathing　Adopt a similar position as for the previous exercise or sit comfortably in a chair where you do not slouch, so leaving your abdominal and chest area open and free. While inhaling and exhaling deeply, concentrate on keeping an even, slow flow throughout. Allow a brief pause after the exhalation before the next breath. This is your moment of complete stillness.

　Both these exercises, because of their rhythmic and expansive nature, induce a state of calm. Practise them whenever you like, for about 10 to 15 minutes, preferably in a quiet place, perhaps in your bedroom before you go to sleep and when you wake.

Diet, exercise, relationships — is the time right for change?
　By scribbling down options in the form of a logic tree (below) it is possible to see where the problems lie; if you wish to make changes, you can now take the first steps!

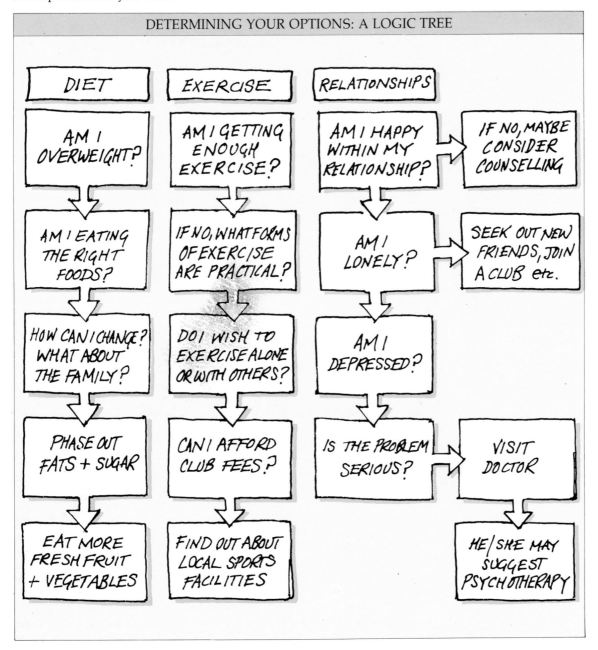

DETERMINING YOUR OPTIONS: A LOGIC TREE

DIET
- AM I OVERWEIGHT?
- AM I EATING THE RIGHT FOODS?
- HOW CAN I CHANGE? WHAT ABOUT THE FAMILY?
- PHASE OUT FATS + SUGAR
- EAT MORE FRESH FRUIT + VEGETABLES

EXERCISE
- AM I GETTING ENOUGH EXERCISE?
- IF NO, WHAT FORMS OF EXERCISE ARE PRACTICAL?
- DO I WISH TO EXERCISE ALONE OR WITH OTHERS?
- CAN I AFFORD CLUB FEES?
- FIND OUT ABOUT LOCAL SPORTS FACILITIES

RELATIONSHIPS
- AM I HAPPY WITHIN MY RELATIONSHIP? → IF NO, MAYBE CONSIDER COUNSELLING
- AM I LONELY? → SEEK OUT NEW FRIENDS, JOIN A CLUB etc.
- AM I DEPRESSED?
- IS THE PROBLEM SERIOUS? → VISIT DOCTOR
- HE/SHE MAY SUGGEST PSYCHOTHERAPY

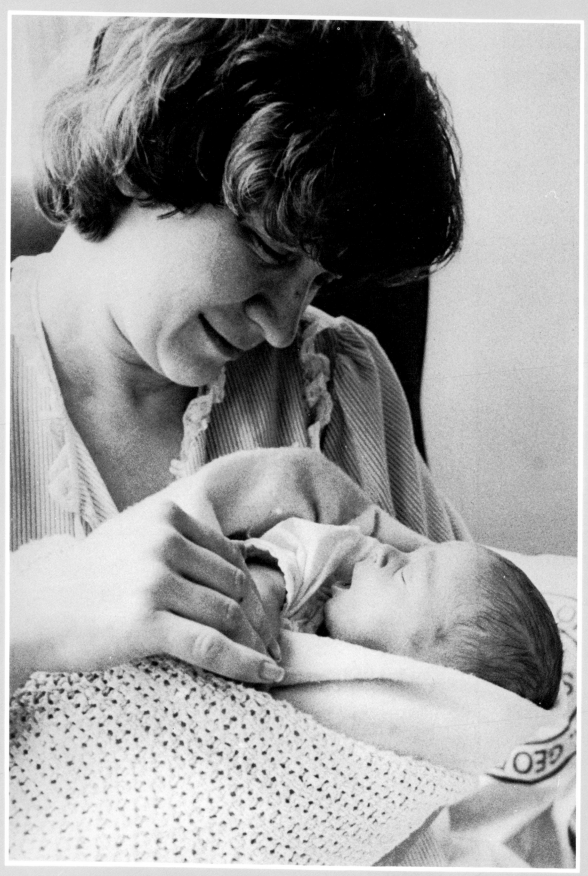

The Fertile Woman

- Preparing for Pregnancy • Fertilization and Pregnancy Testing
- Monitoring your Pregnancy • Ante-Natal Exercises
- Labour and Delivery • After the Birth • Miscarriage
- Abortion • Infertility •

THERE IS NO SUCH THING AS 'A GOOD MOTHER'. There is 'good enough mothering', in paediatrician David Winnicott's famous phrase, and there are happy mothers. Obviously, something is very wrong somewhere if you turn out to be unhappy most of the time, but to expect automatically to become a gloriously happy, efficient and faultless mother from the moment your baby is born is unrealistic. Such paragons do exist, but for most of us mothering is a learning process. The most valuable friends for many women in later life are women they met during pregnancy. And it is usually from other mothers, including your own and your mother-in-law, if you are married, that you begin to learn how to be a mother.

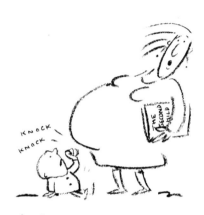

Just as 'good enough mothering' is the best kind, so 'part-time mothering' is a concept that can help to shape your ideas on motherhood. Our society has a tendency to romanticize the relationship between mother and baby, and all of us have a secret longing to be perfect, to provide for our babies consistently, without fatigue and without getting bored or irritable. Indeed, not so very long ago motherhood was considered a full-time job for those not well off enough to employ a nanny. This proved enormously satisfying for some, but the vast majority of women suffered greatly from being tied so restrictively to a young infant, feeling not only resentful and exhausted, but also sensing a loss of their own identity, and guilt for entertaining such 'negative' emotions.

Women *must* think of themselves as human beings first and mothers second. All mothering should be part-time, in the sense that you should maintain your sense of yourself as an individual by taking time off to pursue other interests, to see friends or go to the cinema, or just to relax and read a book. The importance of the father's cooperation in making this possible for you is, of course, paramount. But his role is not just as baby-minder so that you can have some free time. By considering yourself as part of a family team and not a lone captain, you allow the father to establish his own bonding and relationship with the baby. This, in turn, will strengthen your own relationship with father and child, and help mitigate any confusion or resentment the father may be feeling at suddenly having to share your love and attention with a new arrival.

The concept of 'networking' comes to us from the USA. Applied to motherhood it can refer to the family or to a support system of friends and professional helpers. It is important to build such a support system for yourself consciously at this crucial stage in your life. Otherwise, living in large cities or rural areas as many of us do, it is all too easy to become extremely isolated. We no longer take the extended family for granted in the West. Indeed, the emphasis is on getting away from the family home as soon as possible and 'doing one's own thing'. It is now considered almost shameful for a son or daughter to be living at home beyond the age of about 20.

We have gained in some ways from this independence, in defining our own personalities and developing our own interests and direction in life. But we lose in other ways, in terms of the support and understanding we could get from those who have known us from birth and watched and helped us to grow up. Particularly when a woman has her first baby, she often feels great sympathy with, and need for, her own mother. Differences are buried as the two women draw together in a common bond. The support a young mother can gain in this way is extremely valuable, both to her and her child. It is also beneficial for the interrelationship of the generations. For instance, a young child often finds that he or she is better understood by granny than by his or her own parents. Granny is familiar and safe but at one remove from the intense mother/child relationship. Granny may also be at a stage in her life when she has acquired the calm to be tolerant of the demands of a young child.

Of course, things are not always so ideal, and most of us rely greatly on the support of close and caring friends at this time. If, for whatever reasons, you do not have this kind of support, there are organizations that can provide help, or direct you towards a local self-help group (see pages 202/3).

Trusting your own instincts

We live in an age of experts, and many of us become unnerved by what we see as their superior knowledge, distrusting our own instincts and our own experiences. Baby books abound so that young mothers today read avidly the wise words of the specialists, the obstetricians and other gurus. They plan to follow this or that method of birth, and this or that method of feeding and upbringing. Although they may gain many useful tips and feel more secure with this expert knowledge to hand, ultimately only the mother herself knows what it is like to be herself — a mother for the first time, in her own particular circumstances.

Unfortunately, many of us have been educated to distrust, ignore and suppress our instincts. (In fact, eventually — as with all faculties which are not used and cultivated — we may stop having them altogether.) Because Western education has for centuries been dominated by the 'masculine' modes of thought — that is, giving precedence to linear, objective, rational and analytical faculties over subjective, lateral, instinctual and synthesizing faculties — it will probably be at least another generation or two before these more 'feminine' qualities are treated seriously and developed as part of our education. Of course, men and women both have masculine *and* feminine ways of being and thinking within them, to lesser or greater degrees. And just as women are benefiting today from the expression of their 'masculine' side, speaking their minds more, getting responsible jobs and developing their own voices and personalities, so men will (and some already do) benefit from paying attention to their 'feminine' side.

An example of how things are changing quite rapidly is that the concept of lateral thinking — for which women have a particular gift and which used to be downgraded in such cavalier throwaway lines as 'women have grasshopper minds' — has been made into a respectable science now by Edward de Bono. He defined lateral thinking as a thought process in which creative imagination is allowed to have free play and thus possibly hit upon original solutions to what may initially seem difficult or impossible situations. He does not claim, however, that lateral thinking is superior to what he terms 'vertical' thinking — the conventional and unimaginative logical approach. Rather, he argues, the two methods of thinking are complementary.

Of course, the right balance does need to be struck between trusting our own instincts and making use of contemporary scientific findings which can be of advantage to us, but we tend to err on the side of social conditioning and trusting the experts. So bear in mind that what *feels* right for you and your baby most probably *is* right.

Preparing for pregnancy

When you are planning a pregnancy, it is particularly important that you should be aware of your own body, of the foods you eat, of when you have sex, and how you as an individual will respond to being a mother. Such awareness and consequent, informed cooperation with your health-care professionals means you can ensure that you and your baby obtain the best possible care.

First, make sure that you and your partner are in good health, by both paying sensible attention to your diet (pages 74-79). Both of you play your part in the creation of the baby, so you both need to be prepared well in advance for the eventual fertilization.

Planning to conceive

It is important to prepare in this way because no couple can know for sure when they are actually going to conceive; you may not realize for some weeks that you *are* pregnant — yet it is in those first few crucial weeks that your baby's vital organs are being formed.

Stopping contraception   If you have been using an IUD, simply have it removed at the end of a period. You will not need to wait for any bodily adjustment before you start trying to conceive.

If you have been taking any form of contraceptive pill, however, it is best to allow your blood system time to adjust (about three months) before attempting to conceive. In the meantime, use a cap or your partner can use a sheath. Once your menstrual cycle is back to normal it will be easier to

POSSIBLE HAZARDS TO CONCEPTION

Drink, drugs and pregnancy
Even when fertilization has taken place, the egg still has to make its slow progress along one of the Fallopian tubes to the uterus, the journey taking between twelve and eighteen hours. If, however, you are under the influence of alcohol, cannabis or stimulatory or hallucinogenic drugs, or the nicotine of cigarettes, the whole system becomes sluggish and the journey takes much, much longer. The result can be that the egg dies before it can reach the womb, or an ectopic pregnancy may occur, necessitating an emergency operation for its removal. Even if the pregnancy follows the normal pattern, research has shown that the baby of a mother under these influences tends to be lighter at birth, and there is an increased risk of perinatal mortality – death of the baby shortly after birth.

It makes sense, therefore to guard your own health and that of your baby by trying to give up, or at least substantially cut down on, your intake of these stimulants.

Pills and medicines
If you have been in the habit of taking any pills or medicines regularly — for whatever reason — it is sensible to see your doctor before trying to conceive. In the case of a serious condition such as diabetes, it is vitally important anyway that your pregnancy be carefully monitored to ensure that you have the best possible chance of giving birth to a healthy baby.

It is best not to take any pills or medicines either just before or during pregnancy without first consulting your doctor; some pills and medicines can be harmful to

the developing fetus, and can cause birth defects.

Inherited illnesses and abnormalities   If either you or your partner have a relative who suffers from a condition such as haemophilia, cystic fibrosis, spina bifida or Down's syndrome (mongolism), it is important to discuss this with your doctor so that you can have any relevant tests during your ante-natal care. Good medical care while you are pregnant can both lessen the risk of such problems occurring and give early warning so that any necessary additional care can be provided or the possibility of an early abortion can be considered.

The ideas behind natural methods of contraception (see page 25) will help you find out when you are fertile: your temperature dips and then rises on those days when you ovulate, and your cervical mucus becomes free-flowing and stringy.

Record your findings and note the days you make love; when pregnant you will be able to work out the exact time of fertilization.

MONTH																																	
DATE	16	17	18	19	20	21	22	23	24	25	26	27	28	29	30	1	2	3	4	5	6	7	8	9	10	11	12	13	14	15	16		
DAY OF WEEK	T	W	T	F	S	S	M	T	W	T	F	S	S	M	T	W	T	F	S	S	M	T	W	T	F	S	S	M	T	W	T		
DAY OF CYCLE	1	2	3	4	5	6	7	8	9	10	11	12	13	14	15	16	17	18	19	20	21	22	23	24	25	26	27	28	29	30	31	32	33	34
FERTILE PERIOD																																	
SEX		X		X				X					X	X		X		X	X	X	X					X								

(Temperature chart: scale 99.0 down to 98.0 and below, marked .9 .8 .7 .6 .5 .4 .3 .2 .1)

calculate exactly when you are likely to conceive and, once you are pregnant, when your baby will be due.

Likely time for conception   Do not be disappointed if you do not conceive quickly after ceasing to use contraception, particularly if you were using a contraceptive pill. It can take six months or longer; on the other hand you may be lucky and conceive within weeks. Ninety per cent of married couples with no abnormalities should achieve conception within a year, so only after this period is there the slightest cause for concern. Remember, too, that the more anxious you become, the less easy it may be for you to conceive. Relax, and enjoy the novelty of no longer having to worry about contraception!

If, after a year of trying, you have still not become pregnant, it is sensible for you and your partner to see your doctor together and arrange to have tests to establish any possible causes of non-conception. Even if problems are discovered, the situation is by no means dire.

Fertilization

This can be defined as the point when the sperm, having survived its journey through the vagina, the cervix and the body of the uterus, meets the ripe egg and they unite, to form a single cell. The egg's action of bursting out of its follicle in the ovary (see right) is triggered by the entry into the bloodstream of the luteinizing hormone (LH) which is released in mid-cycle. The egg is drawn into the Fallopian tube and is wafted along, aided by the tube's rhythmic contractions; about two thirds of the way down it meets the sperm, usually between seven and twelve hours after sex. Within 48 hours of the cell and sperm meeting a little bundle of cells has been formed which will implant itself in the endometrium — the lining of the womb — and grow into a fetus.

Cigarette smoking has been found to have a particularly deadening effect on the rhythmic action of the Fallopian tubes; one cigarette can stop this action for up to 40 minutes. If you want to conceive, it is advisable not to smoke for five days after sex as this will give the egg time to get into the uterus and begin its development before being destroyed by nicotinic acid.

Pregnancy tests

The earliest, most accurate pregnancy test is a blood test which is done to establish whether or not a hormone called human chorionic gonadotrophin is present in the bloodstream. This is produced by the fertilized ovum and is excreted in the urine. The test — called the beta HCG — can be done privately or some hospitals will perform one but they may only offer to do so if you are one of their patients.

The next most accurate tests come in the form of special kits which can be bought from chemists for a small sum. The kit provides two tests, and will give a positive reading — if you are pregnant — at the point at which your period is between five and seven days late. If the test is negative you should repeat it three to four days later. Quite often anxiety delays your period, and the reassurance of a negative pregnancy test is enough to bring it on.

If you really want to know whether or not you are pregnant you should find out by means of one of the methods outlined above; following the advice of some older doctors, who will tell you to wait until after you have missed your second period, can be catastrophic: by this time the contents of your uterus will have quadrupled in size, your bloodstream will contain a high level of hormones and any decision-making about the outcome will be that much more difficult.

Fertilization is the starting point of all human life. The meeting of the female ovum and the male sperm — each bearing its own load of chromosomes — lays down a unique blueprint for the new individual.

2 Fertilization: millions of sperm enter the woman's body upon ejaculation, but most do not survive the long journey to the uterus. Some 7 to 12 hours after sex the survivors meet up with the ripe ovum. One will manage to break through the 'zona pellucida' or ring of jelly-like cells which surround the ovum. The two sets of chromosomes — 23 each from the ovum and sperm — unite in a single cell, establishing the characteristics of the new child.

3 The fertilized egg grows by the chromosomes integrating and duplicating themselves, a process which will continue until every new cell contains the same set of genetic instructions.

4 Cell division begins on the day after fertilization. At this stage the egg is about 0.2mm in diameter; with each division — or cleavage — it will enlarge.

5 The fertilized egg is wafted down the Fallopian tube by cilia — the mass of tiny hairs that line the tube.

1 The ripe ovum bursts out of its follicle in the ovary and is wafted into the Fallopian tube. The luteinizing hormone (LH) triggers this process at ovulation, midway in the female cycle.

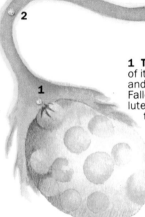

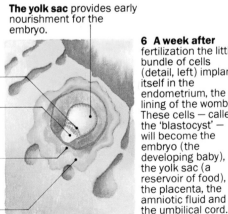

The yolk sac provides early nourishment for the embryo.

The embryo has two layers: the **endoderm** is next to the yolk and the **ectoderm** is next to the amniotic sac.

The amniotic sac

The middle trophoblast layer which later forms the placenta.

The outer trophoblast layer which burrows into the uterus.

6 A week after fertilization the little bundle of cells (detail, left) implants itself in the endometrium, the lining of the womb. These cells — called the 'blastocyst' — will become the embryo (the developing baby), the yolk sac (a reservoir of food), the placenta, the amniotic fluid and the umbilical cord.

113

The stages of pregnancy

The first seven weeks of pregnancy When the fertilized egg, having implanted itself in the nourishing wall of the womb, has grown to around half a million cells, specific substances called 'auxins' can be detected. These organize the development of the embryo into the various parts of the body — backbone, arms, legs and internal organs.

This is the most vulnerable time in the whole of human existence, so it is absolutely crucial that a mother-to-be is particularly attentive to her health care during this period. In the early 1960s there was an appalling epidemic of babies born with either deformed arms and legs or none at all, following the use of the drug Thalidomide in a sleeping pill prescribed to insomniac pregnant women. The drug was withdrawn, but it is especially important not to take any drugs or medicines of any kind during these first seven-and-a-half weeks: common cold remedies, herbal medications and smoking have all been implicated in of birth defects.

Other serious problems can arise if, at this time, the mother is deficient in folic acid or other essential vitamins and minerals, or if the mother contracts German measles during this period. However on the subject of vitamins, we do not know what mega-doses or even small additional doses of vitamins may do to a growing fetus so try to follow your instincts and advice you really *trust*.

Eight to fourteen weeks During this very early stage of pregnancy the majority of women experience malaise and nausea. Although biologically a woman's body is 'programmed' to carry and give birth to a baby, there is a very real sense in which her body is greatly upset by the rapid hormonal changes which take place during pregnancy. She may experience either 'morning sickness' (which can in fact last all day), 'emotional lability' (sitting on the bathroom floor dissolved in tears), clumsiness, lack of appetite, cravings for specific foods, or a combination of all of these reactions.

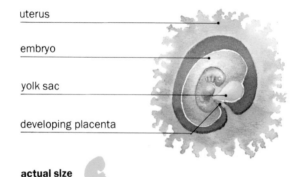

uterus

embryo

yolk sac

developing placenta

actual size

Within two weeks of conception, the ball of cells, or 'blastocyst', has firmly rooted itself to the uterine wall and begins to fold into layers that will become the baby's body systems.

By the fourth week of pregnancy, the embryo (left) has the essential foundations for a nervous system (ectoderm), a digestive system (endoderm) and a

blood system (mesoderm). The embryo has a definite head and tail.

The spinal cord and brain have developed from the neural tube, the heart is already beating and some of the rudimentary blood vessels are joining together to form the umbilical cord that will provide the life-support line from mother to baby.

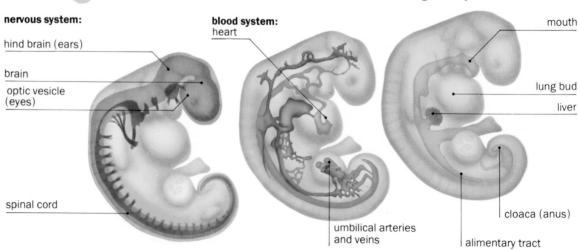

nervous system:

hind brain (ears)

brain

optic vesicle (eyes)

spinal cord

blood system:
heart

umbilical arteries and veins

digestive system:

mouth

lung bud

liver

cloaca (anus)

alimentary tract

Fortunately, vitamin B$_6$ supplements can do much to alleviate these symptoms. Check this possibility with your clinic or doctor.

A positive attitude in the knowledge that these symptoms are signs of a healthy pregnancy and a properly growing baby can help a mother to get through this period. These hormonal changes are in fact the body's way of reminding you that you are pregnant and should take care of yourself and, far from being a source of worry, are perfectly normal.

From twelve to thirty-two weeks After 12 weeks, and up to 32 weeks, although your abdomen becomes increasingly large the chances are you will probably feel absolutely marvellous. Most women experience an increase in energy at this time and find themselves enjoying all the 'nesting' activities of preparation for the baby's arrival — shopping, decorating and so on.

From thirty-two to forty weeks These last two months should be a relaxing time while you await delivery. If you have been working you should have given up by now; if you feel energetic enough to carry on do so, but don't push yourself too hard. It is particularly important to continue to eat well; don't worry about gaining weight as you will lose this once the baby is born.

Some women may be affected by high blood pressure throughout pregnancy; if this has been the case it is during these last two months that weekly — or even twice weekly — visits to the hospital for it to be checked may be necessary. If the problem is particularly severe short or longer stays in hospital may be requested. Some women claim that this 'toing and froing' from the hospital exacerbates the problem! Relaxation and rest should help and, as high blood pressure can be brought on by anxiety, talking over your worries — with the medical staff, other mothers or your antenatal teacher, should be reassuring.

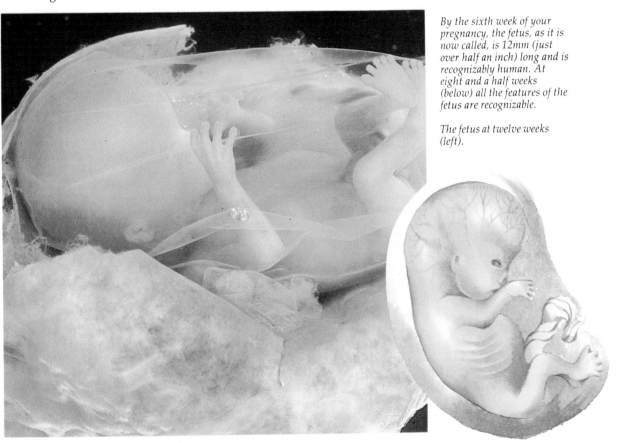

By the sixth week of your pregnancy, the fetus, as it is now called, is 12mm (just over half an inch) long and is recognizably human. At eight and a half weeks (below) all the features of the fetus are recognizable.

The fetus at twelve weeks (left).

MONITORING YOUR PREGNANCY

There are certain tests and procedures that will be reassuring to you during pregnancy and will safeguard the health of your baby, and yourself. These are:

BLOOD TESTS

Rubella (German measles) Ideally, you should make sure that you are immune to rubella *before* you become pregnant. Your doctor can give you a blood test and if the results show that you are not immune, you can have a simple vaccination — after which you should avoid pregnancy for three months. If you catch rubella while pregnant, especially during the first three months when your baby's organs, muscles, limbs and bones are forming, it can do severe damage to the baby's heart and nervous system and cause deafness and blindness. It may also cause miscarriage or still birth.

Early in pregnancy you will be routinely tested for rubella and if you are not then immune, you will probably be offered immunization after your baby is born. If you are given immunization, it is important that you do not become pregnant again within three months of the injection.

If, during pregnancy, you are not immune and accidentally come into contact with someone who has rubella, tell your doctor without delay. Blood tests will show whether you have been infected and if this is the case you should consider an abortion.

Haemoglobin level The proportion of red pigment in the blood, which carries oxygen round the body, is checked. If this level is too low, you are anaemic and

your baby may not grow properly. However, by detecting anaemia at an early stage in pregnancy it is possible to correct it by relatively simple treatment such as taking specially prescribed iron supplement tablets.

Rhesus status Everybody is either rhesus negative or rhesus positive, and it is important that your rhesus status and whether or not you have antibodies against the other are both checked out early in pregnancy:
- If you are a rhesus negative woman having a child by a rhesus negative man, there is no problem: your baby will be rhesus negative and you will not make antibodies.
- If you are a rhesus positive mother having a child by a rhesus positive man, in the same way there is no problem.
- However, if you are a rhesus negative mother, with a rhesus positive partner, and have had either a child together before, or a transfusion or an abortion, you might already possess antibodies against your own baby if he or she is rhesus positive. (If the baby is rhesus negative this will not happen. It is the antibodies complication that makes it important to know your blood group before you plan a pregnancy.) Even if mother and child are of different groups, modern medical techniques ensure that no one suffers. The formation of antibodies can be prevented in the majority of cases by an anti-D vaccine called Rhogam.

Other blood tests which are useful for mothers of certain ethnic origins. For

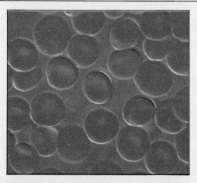

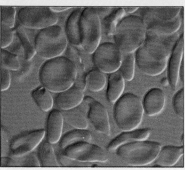

Slides of blood cells as seen through the microscope. Normal red cells appear as well-rounded discs (top). In sickle cell anaemia (below) the cells are distorted, some taking on an oblong shape.

instance, Jewish parents may be tested for Tay Sachs disease (which causes blindness). If you are of black African origin you will be tested for sickle cell anaemia, which causes failure to grow, joint pain and haemorrhages. If you or your partner come from the Mediterranean area, it is a sensible precaution to be tested for thalassaemia (which causes problems similar to sickle cell anaemia).

The spina bifida test This measures the alphafetoprotein level in your blood and can detect certain abnormalities in the development of the baby's central nervous system. *It is crucial that this test is done at 16 weeks.* If the test is positive — if, that is, it shows that your baby is causing an excess of this substance — you will be asked to undergo amniocentesis, to measure the actual amount of alphafetoprotein in the fluid surrounding the baby. At the same time a complete fetal anatomy ultrasound scan is generally used to show whether or not your baby's spine is developing normally. If the brain or spinal cord is not normal, your obstetrician will discuss with you whether or not you might wish to have the pregnancy terminated.

URINE TESTS

Urine tests are best done on a sample passed first thing in the morning, for at this time it is most concentrated. The tests are for a number of things, but the most important are as follows:

Presence of sugar in urine
It is not unusual for pregnant women to have sugar in their urine from time to time, but if it recurs repeatedly, you will be checked for the possible presence of diabetes. If the test proves positive, you will receive greater vigilance to ensure that any sign of abnormality in your baby is detected at a very early stage.

Presence of protein in urine In early pregnancy this warns of a possible urinary tract infection. In later pregnancy it could be an indication of toxaemia, a condition that sends poisonous substances through the body via the bloodstream. In either event, appropriate treatment can be given.

If you have any other possible problems on your mind when you go for the early tests, jot them down so that there is no possibility of forgetting them in the flurry of tests. The earlier you raise such issues, the sooner you can be reassured or given any necessary attention.

WOMB TESTS

Amniocentesis For mothers in their thirties it is sensible to consider amniocentesis for the detection of Down's syndrome. Amniocentesis simply involves carefully withdrawing some of the fluid surrounding the baby for the purpose of tests. Usually, this takes place at about 16 weeks, by which stage all the major organs of the baby are fully formed. As the doctor checks through ultrasound to see that it is safe to insert the needle in preparation for drawing off some of the fluid, it is sometimes possible to see the baby sucking her thumb or, if it is a boy, the genital organs may be quite obvious.

During amniocentesis you lie close by the ultrasound machine and on the TV monitor can actually see your baby moving about. After the doctor has administered a local anaesthetic, you can perhaps also watch the needle being inserted in between the placenta and the baby and thus be visually reassured that this does not bother the baby at all. When the needle is removed, the tiny puncture hole will be covered with a plaster and it is sensible to rest ▶

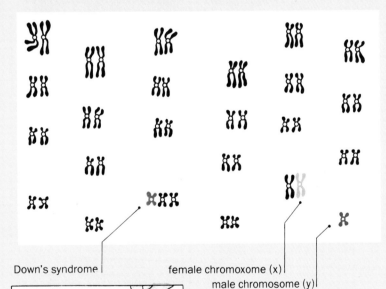

Down's syndrome

female chromoxome (x)
male chromosome (y)

In amniocentesis (left) fluid is drawn off from around the baby so that it can be examined for genetic defects. Every cell in the body contains chromosomes (above); these carry all the genetic information which will determine the characteristics of the individual.

It is normal to have 46 chromosomes arranged in pairs: in Down's syndrome (mongolism), however, each cell has an extra bit of chromosome material (circled). This is called a chromosomal trisomy.

as much as possible during the next 24 hours. Meanwhile the valuable amniotic fluid is taken off for the various necessary tests.

Chorionic biopsy Around the world doctors and scientists are always evaluating new procedures for trying to prevent birth defects or to diagnose birth defects as soon as possible, so that the parents do have the choice of early termination or, in rare cases, intra-uterine treatment.

Chorionic biopsy is one such new procedure; it can be performed as early as 12 weeks from the beginning of pregnancy and involves putting a tiny tube in through the cervix and removing some cells from the baby's tissues. From these cells, many of the tests that could later be done on the amniotic fluid can be done at this much earlier stage in pregnancy (if these cells grow well in tissue culture). At the moment, the technique is still experimental, but indications are that it will be a very useful new procedure.

Ultrasound At between 12 to 16 weeks your baby will be large enough for any fetal abnormalities to be detected, so at this stage you may have an ultrasound check. This is an essential test for mothers aged over 35, particularly if they and the father both smoke, for the statistics for fetal heart defects are 46 in 1,000. It is often recommended that high risk mothers have ultrasound scans at 8 to 9 weeks, 15 to 16 weeks, 28 weeks and 36 weeks.

As far as is known at present there is nothing to fear from ultrasound.

Some babies respond to ultrasound and others do not. We now know that from about 16 weeks the baby can recognize and distinguish the sound of its mother's voice from others, responding with increased activity and raised metabolic reactions. Similarly, some babies get quite excited, responding by shifting around the womb in a spate of activity when the ultrasound equipment is directed onto them. This is not surprising: mice communicate with their young through ultrasound and we know that there are many high frequencies of noise which we, as adults, do not hear but which may be audible within the womb.

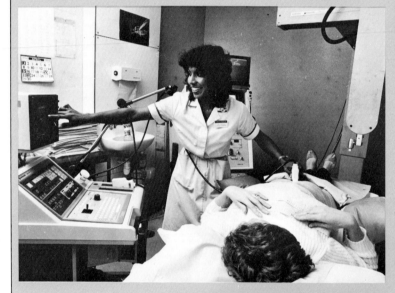

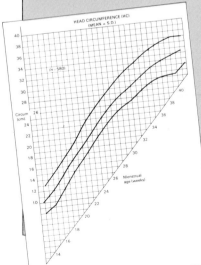

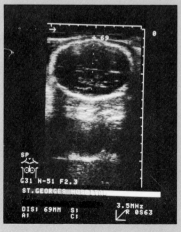

The use of ultrasound equipment (left) gives medical staff the great advantage of being able to monitor accurately the growth of the unborn baby.

Measurements are recorded on a graph (far left), while the x-ray picture (right) shows the size of the baby's head.

Recent research work has indicated patterns of growth in normal and slow-growing babies; if a baby is not making good progress, it may be delivered before full term. Human babies have an enormous potential for growth; once out of the womb, and possibly in a special care unit, the baby will catch up rapidly.

Preparing for labour and birth

The best training for any sort of hard work is to get fit — super-fit sportswomen usually have easy and trouble-free labours and births. This is in part because they are familiar with the limits to which they can take their bodies. They feel in control and, having crossed the pain threshhold many times during training, are not frightened by the pain they now experience in labour. They remain relaxed and alert, and do not panic, and this has the effect of greatly reducing any pain, in that pain is exacerbated by fear and tension. Certainly, therefore, the best training for the hard, physical labour of giving birth is to get fit before pregnancy.

It should be emphasized, however, that any pregnant woman who attempts a regime of aerobic-type exercises (even if she has previously done so with no ill effects) may put herself and her baby at risk. Gentle relaxation and stretching exercises are the ideal. Also, if you have any medical problem you would be wise to discuss the question of appropriate exercise with your obstetrician before you begin.

The specific training for labour, so that the mother is familiar with her own body and what she is going to experience, should begin at least 10 weeks before her baby is due. There are excellent courses run by the National Childbirth Trust, but many large hospitals organize free classes for both mothers and fathers.

When you are planning a pregnancy you have to make three basic decisions:
- Where will you have your baby?
- Which specific training do you wish to do for labour and birth?
- Which type of analgesic or anaesthesia may you need during labour?

Where you will have your baby While the choice is basically between having your baby at home or in hospital there are other options: finding a birth centre (these are now being set up in some areas), or opting for 'shared care' where your doctor and midwives attend to you in a unit which is part of a maternity wing in hospital.

Home confinement A recent study, conducted in the Oxfordshire area, found that 92 per cent of the women questioned would choose to have their babies in the familiar surroundings of their own homes. Since the mechanization of birth in the 1950s and the accompanying increase in medical control, most births have taken place in hospital where doctors often have charge rather than the mother.

While many women fully intend, at the onset of pregnancy, to opt for a home confinement they are often dissuaded: sometimes for medical reasons but, very often, because of the disinclination of their own doctor. However, the situation is changing and mothers-to-be are having a greater say.

A very positive aspect of home delivery is that birth becomes a social event with your partner, members of your family and friends giving you help and encouragement in your labour. However, a home confinement will almost certainly be inadvisable if you fall into any of the following categories:
- If you have previously had an abnormal labour.
- If you are under 17 or over 42 (in which case the chances of needing a Caesarian section are between 50 and 60 per cent).
- If you have already had four pregnancies (often the first is also considered more risky).
- If you are under-nourished, over-tired or not in good health.

Practical help and advice on arranging a home confinement can be obtained from both the Maternity Alliance and the Association of Radical Midwives (see pages 202/23).

A good alternative to giving birth at home is to find a birth centre. The staff

Where you will have your baby

Your choices in childbirth

ANTE-NATAL EXERCISES

Regular exercise during pregnancy will help you get into shape for the hard work of labour and delivery. Your pelvic and abdominal muscles are the most important and toning them up will help support the growing baby and make childbirth easier. As well as carrying out these exercises, you should also attend ante-natal classes.

Take it slowly and build up gradually — if anything hurts unduly, consult your ante-natal teacher.

Sit cross-legged with pillows in the small of your back for support. Circle your head clockwise and anti-clockwise, breathing deeply.

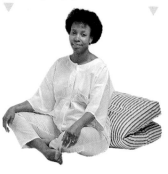

With your hands on your shoulders lean to one side then to the other. Feel the stretch down each side.

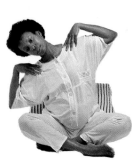

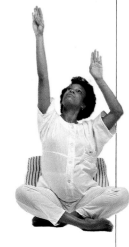

For sleeping/relaxing: lie with a pillow to support your abdomen. Draw one knee up and rest it on the pillow. Your lower arm can support your head.

With your shoulders relaxed lift both arms above your head. Stretch one arm to the ceiling then the other. Look up at your outstretched hand.

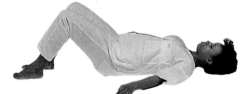

Lie on your back, knees bent, the small of your back pressing into the floor. Bring the soles of your feet together, let your knees fall outwards and bounce them gently.

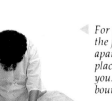

For pelvis and thighs: sit on the floor with your legs apart. Lean forward and place your hands in front of you. Curve your back and bounce gently.

For thighs and pelvis: stand with your feet slightly apart. Raise your arms in front. Slowly bend your knees and crouch as low as you can and squat. Use a chair for support if necessary.

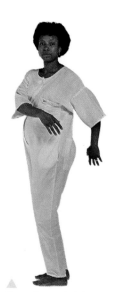

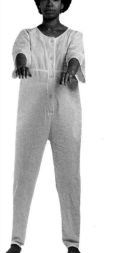

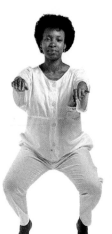

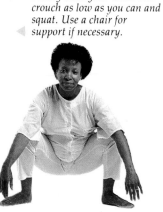

For spine and abdomen: stand with your feet apart and your arms by your sides. Keep your feet still and twist gently, first to the left and then to the right. Ease up if your lower back hurts.

are predominantly female and the atmosphere aims to be as 'homely' as possible. While everything is done to ensure that the woman in labour is having a happy, social time, back-up services are on hand.

Hospital birth   The overwhelming majority of women give birth in hospital; one particularly positive aspect of a hospital confinement, compared to home, is the definite protocol and acceptance of the fact of birth — even in the most enlightened family the reaction of other members of the family to the labouring woman can be upsetting. But.as far as choosing the hospital goes, there is no substitute for good local information: consult your friends and neighbours about their experiences and ask your doctor's advice. While you do have the right of referral to any hospital you choose, bear in mind such practical considerations as its location — a long bus or car journey for ante-natal visits could be very inconvenient.

The most important thing about having your baby in hospital is to make sure you have somebody with you — your partner, a woman friend or a member of your family — to give you help and encouragement. While everyone in the obstetric team is generally prepared to do their utmost for you and your baby, their overriding concern will be for the baby and so it is important to have someone there concentrating on your needs and helping you decide on suggested procedures.

Having your baby in hospital may well ensure a pain-free labour because of the availability of anaesthetics; additionally such measures as monitoring of the baby's heart-beat will take place. You may well be given intravenous fluids to stop you from becoming dehydrated and to keep your strength up during labour, and these can be very helpful. In a rare emergency — for example extreme fatigue on the part of the mother or the baby — there is the possibility of a Caesarian section.

A variation on hospital birth which is increasingly available is 'shared care', where you are looked after by midwives together with your own, or another, doctor. Labour and delivery take place in hospital, with all the back-up facilities; because your doctor knows your whole circumstances, you and your baby — if there are no complications — may be allowed home after six hours. The philosophy behind this care is less reliant on technology and routine procedure; inductions are rarely performed, but, should there be an emergency, all the facilities of the hospital are available.

Over and above deciding on any particular method for giving birth is the importance of establishing understanding and trust between mother, father (or whoever will be with you at the birth) and the midwife and obstetrician. This is fundamental to the essentially cooperative nature of the birth process and sets the scene for a positive experience.

Natural childbirth   This is birth unimpeded by drugs or machinery of any sort. However, natural childbirth when the mother's pelvis is too small or where the baby is in a wrong and potentially dangerous position could result in the death of both mother and baby. It is important for all mothers who decide that they wish to remain in control of their labours to understand exactly what the risks are for them and their babies.

Some hospitals encourage this method, some do not. In those that do, there will be all the necessary equipment standing by just in case anything should go wrong. At King's College Hospital, in London, of the 40 per cent of patients who elect for natural childbirth, only about a quarter of them actually go through with it. But in Glasgow, where the maternity wing is run by midwives practically all of whom are women, the birth is a truly cooperative venture; about 50 per cent of mothers opt for natural childbirth and about 70 per cent of them are able to complete the birth in this way.

Much depends on the previous experience of the doctors and the midwives,

How you will have your baby

121

and whether they can be happy taking part in a cooperative birth or feel that they need to be in control at all times. A study of maternal deaths in any Western country shows that giving birth is not always a benign and serene and safe process for either mother or baby, but certainly for well over 80 per cent of women in Britain this is the case.

Active childbirth　This simply involves undertaking a training programme for contraction awareness and control so that the delivery happens in the optimum time without side effects on you or your baby. Advocates of active childbirth recommend standing, kneeling or squatting to relieve the pain of labour. The theory overlaps with that of natural childbirth, both of which emphasize the active participation of the woman and her partner during labour and delivery. It is an advisable training for all pregnant women and if your hospital does not provide them, seek out good antenatal classes through the Maternity Alliance or National Childbirth Trust.

Leboyer method　Leboyer believes that the first, anguished cry of the newborn often provoked by a slap on the back from midwife or obstetrician, is entirely unnecessary. It is, he claims, the terrified protest of a bewildered and exhausted baby, for whom birth is quite difficult and momentous enough without the accompaniment of loud voices, bright lights, cold hands and steely equipment, and above all, insensitive handling by medical staff.

The Leboyer method of delivery uses every technique to reduce stress to mother and child: soft, dimmed lights and a warm, cosy atmosphere where staff talk in whispers or work in total silence. When the baby is born, it is immediately placed gently on the mother's abdomen. And, contrary to regular hospital practice, the umbilical cord is not cut straight away–which act, Leboyer maintains, provokes in the baby a terrified sense of imminent suffocation and death, hence the first gasping inhalation and wail of anguish. Instead, the cord is allowed to continue pulsating (sometimes for as long as five minutes or more) until the natural switchover mechanism from cord to lungs takes place of its own accord.

Michel Odent method　By June 1983, Michel Odent, chief obstetrician at Pithiviers Hospital in France, had conducted his one-hundredth delivery under water. His birthing pool has now become well known and is being tried elsewhere, but is still difficult to find in this country. Akin to Leboyer in his attitudes regarding the importance of the birth experience for child and mother, and the warm, reassuring atmosphere that should surround the event, Odent does not advise but offers his pool to mothers as something they might like to try during labour. The temperature of the water is 37°C (98°F) and the dimensions of the pool are two metres (six and a half feet) in diameter and deep enough to allow the woman to change position as she may wish.

Odent believes that the pool facilitates the first stage of labour because of the reduced secretion of noradrenaline and other catecholamines by this method. Also, the effect of water on the nerves, the muscles and on vascular action is to help to ease any tension, pressure or pain the woman might be experiencing. On a psychological level he has found that even just seeing and hearing the water have an effect on the woman's inhibitions and anxiety, relaxing her and encouraging her to cry out and go with her contractions.

Most of the births do not actually happen under water but some do. There is no danger whatever to the infant, however, because the first inhalation and cry are triggered by contact with air. The mother gives birth in a kneeling position and the newborn child is placed immediately in her arms, allowing instant eye and touch contact. Contrary to current popular practise, however, Odent does not encourage the father to be present at the birth. He believes birth is a female experience and that an anxious father may well transmit his nerves to the already labouring mother.

Every pregnant woman hopes that her baby will be born within a few hours and with no complications. However, every mother-to-be should be aware of the difficulties which *can* occur and how she and her partner, her midwife and her doctor, can make the best decisions, and make them at the right time, so that her baby is born healthy.

For a hospital birth, when you first visit the hospital where your baby is to be born, an experienced midwife will show you the labour bed, the labour chair and/or the labour pool. She will discuss your preferences and will probably give you a leaflet detailing the various methods of obtaining pain relief in labour. On this latter consideration, Professor Norman Morris of the Charing Cross Hospital has a very useful and encouraging piece of advice to offer: 'Just remember you will only have one labour pain at a time and most people can cope with one of anything at a time.'

Gas and air machine You and your partner will both be taught how to use this before labour.

Injections of analgesic drugs These are individually calculated for each woman and are administered by the midwife.

Epidural anaesthesia Midway through your pregnancy you and your obstretician will discuss what type of analgesic you may prefer and most centres will now provide epidurals if needed. In your discussion with the obstetrician, ask for an explanation of the possible complications, all of which

Analgesia in childbirth

PREPARING FOR THE BIRTH

Hospital confinement
You can save yourself any possibility of last minute panic or stress by putting the following items into a bag or case two or three weeks before the due date. (Labour can commence unexpectedly early.)
● Two night-dresses, front-opening if you intend to breast-feed.
● Dressing gown and slippers.
● Nursing bras if you intend to breast-feed; otherwise, any good supportive bras.
● Six to eight pairs of cotton briefs to hold sanitary towels in place. You will have a discharge for several weeks after the birth, so towels are essential. The hospital may provide these, as well as nappies and most items for the immediate care of your baby. But do not depend on this; check in advance.
● Towels with adhesive strips will be more comfortable than those that have to be looped on to a sanitary belt, so you may prefer to buy this

particular type anyway.
● Toiletries: sponge or six to eight flannels, toothbrush and paste, mild soap, sachet of shampoo, brush and comb.
● A second bag could be prepared with items for when you come out of hospital, containing clothes for yourself and baby clothes, plus a baby shawl or blanket.
● Also, make a list of the phone numbers of your hospital, local ambulance service, doctor or midwife, and keep them either by your telephone or with the appropriate coins for your nearest telephone-box.

Home confinement
Your midwife will visit you at about 32 weeks to discuss arrangements for the birth, and the room. This need not be the bedroom; you could use a sitting-room or any room which is most comfortable and has the best access to hot water. Some weeks before the due date the midwife will leave a pack of all the sterile items

that are necessary. In addition you will need the following:
● Low bed (without a footboard) or mattress on the floor.
● Low chair.
● Packs of sanitary towels.
● Antiseptic solution.
● A large bowl to receive the placenta.
● A graded jug for measuring blood loss after delivery.
● Clock or watch with a second hand to time contractions.
● Ice cube chips for the mother to suck, plus a fine spray to refresh her.
● A small flanelette sheet or shawl in which to wrap the baby.
● Plenty of plastic sheets or newspapers to deal with the amount of blood produced (usually 2 pints).
● Disposable waste bags for soiled towels.
● A hot-water bottle in case the mother gets cold.
● A camera if you want to take photographs or even a video film.

can be remedied providing that you have the immediate, skilled attention of the anaesthetist. Check that if you have an epidural you will also have this skilled monitoring available. The epidural is administered via a small plastic tube, inserted close by, but not into the spinal canal; an anaesthetic dose is administered half-way through labour, and topped up by the midwife as needed. An epidural numbs only the area of the body causing pain, and leaves the mother alert and able to participate actively in the birth.

Indications that labour has begun

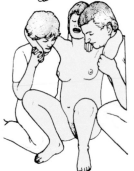

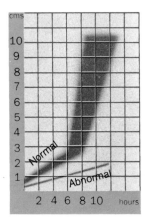

The best birth position is the one that is comfortable. Squatting is the most efficient position for using gravity.

Labour

Towards the end of pregnancy, every so often you will put a hand on your abdomen and find that the whole area is rock-hard. This is painless rehearsal for labour and it is a good idea when you are sitting down watching television or lying in bed to put a hand flat across the middle of your stomach and observe the gradual tightening, then slackening of the uterus. Usually, the day before going into labour proper you will feel these sensations frequently, and, in between these contractions, you will also feel lots of fetal activity as your baby prepares for its birth.

When you are in true labour you become very aware of these contractions. For the first three to four hours, contractions are between 15 to 20 minutes apart and last for about one to two minutes or so. Throughout labour the contractions get closer and closer together and more and more intense. Time them, because with your first baby it is sensible to go to hospital when they are about ten minutes apart.

Before going into hospital, have something to eat — you will need all your energy. But do not have a heavy meal, particularly anything rich. Your stomach will not be able to cope with digesting a large amount of food at this point. Eat light foods: yoghurt, fruit, some wholemeal toast or biscuits, perhaps with fruit juice.

The duration of labour   Some 50 per cent of labours start off with a slight bleeding or pinkish discharge, then during labour the 'bag' of membrane in which the baby has lived so far finally ruptures, and a flood of amniotic fluid is released. Some labours actually initiate like this, and if this 'breaking of the waters' happens while you are out or during the night, it is sensible to go straight to hospital.

The uterus contracts in order to push the baby out in a natural, rhythmic movement that occurs spontaneously during the birth process. However, babies vary greatly in how much effort it takes to push them out. The process can involve as few as 50 to 60 contractions or as many as 200.

Modern labours should not last longer than between six to twelve hours because, at the end of that time, maternal fatigue may well be compounded by fetal distress. If labour has reached this point, your midwife and obstetrician will decide on the best course of action, which may (for example), be a Caesarian section. There are, however, some women who have a somewhat desultory or intermittent labour process that can last for one to two days before enough 'work' is done to ensure the safe arrival of the baby.

Most midwives, and some obstetricians, by the time they have completed their training can detect quite early on abnormal patterns of labour.

Birth positions   Each pregnant woman finds ways of sitting and lying that are comfortable for her. Being in labour is no different. Some women prefer to lie down, some prefer to crouch — the downward pull of gravity in this position helps the contractions, and you can be supported by a birthing chair or stool. (Some medical museums exhibit examples of what they label 'birthing stools'. In fact, these are so near to the ground that were they indeed to be used by the pregnant woman she would have a very bad time. They were intended for, and used by, the attendants at the birth!)

Friedman curves *plot cervical widening, or dilatation, on a graph during labour. If dilatation is not within normal limits the midwife and obstetrician will analyse the woman's progress.*

124

The position of the baby in the womb prior to labour can influence the sort of birth you have. The most common position is the cephalic presentation in which the part of the baby that will be born first — the presenting part — is the head. If the baby is in the breech position (buttocks first), the doctor will give you a pelvic examination to determine whether or not the baby should be delivered by Caesarian section. If the baby is in the cephalic position but facing forward (posterior presentation — right), the bony skull will press against your sacrum and this can cause back pain and result in an erratic and prolonged labour.

During the last four weeks of pregnancy, the presenting part engages in the pelvic cavity ready for birth. When labour starts — no one knows quite why — the tough, fibrous cervix must first soften and thin out, a process known as effacement. Uterine contractions then continue to widen the cervix.

This is called dilatation of the cervix and it is measured in centimetres — at ten centimetres (four inches) the cervix is said to be fully dilated. You are then at the end of the first stage of labour and ready to push the baby out into the world. Medical staff will calculate the extent of dilatation by internal examination at regular intervals throughout your labour.

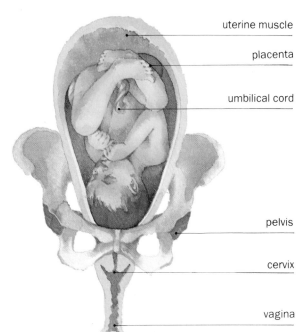

uterine muscle

placenta

umbilical cord

pelvis

cervix

vagina

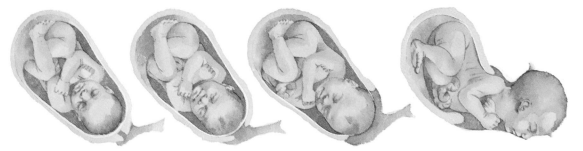

During effacement the cervix thins out and is drawn up around the baby's head. Pushing at this stage may damage the cervix.

When effacement is complete, further contractions dilate the cervix. You can now help your baby on its way by pushing.

When the cervix is fully dilated, the baby moves down through the pelvis. A mirror will allow you to see your baby's head.

The head rotates so that the baby is born facing the mother's rectum. It turns again to the side before the shoulders and body are born.

Your partner will be of great help to you during labour, acting, in a way, as a 'birth coach'. In the early stages he can keep you company and give you reassurance. As the contractions get stronger, in the second stage, he will be able to help you change position and encourage you to practise your breathing and relaxation techniques. And, finally, he will be able to describe what is happening, and will be with you to welcome your new baby into the world.

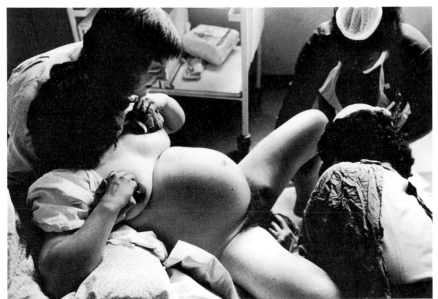

Delivery

The first and most important rule of giving birth is that every woman should have someone with her from the moment that she enters the birth room. This may sound an obvious point, but it is worthwhile to stress it — remembering that the doctors, midwives and obstetricians may all be evidently concerned principally for the baby's safety and well-being. It is all too easy for the mother to come to feel forgotten, ignored or just a machine for giving birth. Many women report feeling terrible depression and fear, in large part due to the sheer exhaustion of giving birth. So it is crucial to have your partner, or husband, by your side caring for your needs — if he is not available, make sure a friend or relative is with you. But your partner's presence is really ideal — he can describe for you what is happening and give you loving encouragement and support. He will also share with you that triumphant and tender moment when your newly-born child is first handed to you.

Episiotomy

It is a tradition in some hospitals that, just as the head is about to emerge (crowning), the nurse or obstetrician makes a cut into the vaginal tissues (called an episiotomy), through the muscle tissue around the opening of the vagina to assist delivery. In recent years this automatic enlarging of the vaginal opening has been increasingly questioned, for the grounds on which an episiotomy was originally performed – among others, to prevent a prolapse in the mother – are actually indefensible. If a prolapse (that is, the collapsing of the uterus is going to happen, it will have happened *before* this stage. In any case the perineal muscles are not involved in supporting the uterus.

Another factor against automatic episiotomy is that scar tissue resulting from hasty sewing up of the cut can cause trouble later. Contrary to popular belief, torn tissues heal naturally and smoothly. However, there is no reason for the perineum to tear if the right preventive techniques are employed: depending on the training of the midwife present, a perineal massage is more effective than a routine episiotomy in the majority of cases. Perineal massage involves the midwife inserting her hand into the vagina some time before the baby begins the descent into the birth canal, in order to massage the pelvic muscles with her fingers. This relaxes the vagina and causes it to be so well lubricated that the baby slides out almost always without tearing, removing any need for episiotomy.

An episiotomy becomes essential, however, if there is to be a forceps delivery or any other need for manipulation of the baby. It is carried out under these circumstances to prevent a tear into the rectum. Before the introduction of antibiotics such a tear commonly resulted in a fistula (tiny opening between the rectum and vagina) and chronic ill-health for years.

Forceps

The delivery of babies by forceps is constantly controversial. Without doubt forceps deliveries have achieved as much good as they have harm. The commonest indication for a straightfoward forceps delivery in modern obstetrics is maternal fatigue or exhaustion. This type of delivery is most usually carried out at the end of the second stage of labour. There should be no force used — the forceps are designed to make it impossible to crush the baby's head and the procedure should be a gentle lifting out of the head and body from the vaginal passage.

Much more controversial are the forceps used in higher extraction techniques; these should always be carried out by the most experienced obstetrician available, after an explanation and effective anaesthesia have been given to the mother.

Breech births

A breech birth is when the baby is facing bottom first or down, rather than head down. The baby can be delivered either with special extraction techniques or by Caesarian section. It can be a great disappointment to a young, healthy mother who has trained for an active birth to be told at 36 weeks that her baby is a 'breech' and it will be safer therefore to have a Caesarian. Whether or not she *is* thus advised will depend on the training and experience of her obstetrics team, and until the safety rates for breech deliveries in various hospitals are made available to us it is sensible for each individual mother to accept — after due explanation and reassurance — the method that works best in that particular hospital.

It is a tradition in some hospitals that, just as the head is about to emerge (crowning), the nurse or obstetrician makes a cut into the vaginal tissues (called an episiotomy), through the muscle tissue around the opening of the vagina to assist delivery. In recent years this automatic enlarging of the vaginal opening has been increasingly questioned, for the grounds on which an episiotomy was originally performed – among others, to prevent a prolapse in the mother – are actually indefensible. If a prolapse (that is, the collapsing of the uterus is going to happen, it will have happened *before* this stage. In any case the perineal muscles are not involved in supporting the uterus.

Caesarian section

For the last ten years, since the advent of safe epidural anaesthesia, having a baby by Caesarian has become a much less frightening prospect for both mother and father. If you know in advance that it is to take place, you will go into hospital at the appointed time and, once in the operating theatre, will be painted with an antiseptic from armpits to thighs (many women comment on the coldness of the solution — so be warned!). However, the epidural inserted then at the base of your spine should cause little discomfort. Some hospitals still favour a general anaesthetic, regarding it as better for both mother and baby. An incision is then made into your abdomen and, if you wish, you can watch the whole procedure without fear of feeling any pain. At the moment of delivery you will feel a tremendous pressure under your rib cage rather than in the abdomen, as the uterus is pulled down and the baby scooped out. The baby will be given to you immediately for a brief greeting, then you can relax and sleep while the incision is stitched and you are taken back to your ward.

Some obstetricians allow the father to take a home video of the proceedings, thus providing a positive memory of a happy and satisfying event. Remember, as long as you are delivered of a healthy baby, you don't *have* to give birth 'naturally' to experience the momentous occasion of birth.

Induction

This is when labour is triggered artificially by the obstetrician. After a discussion with her, you will probably be asked to come into hospital the night before or very early on the morning of the planned birth.

Labour is induced by one of two methods: by synthetic pituitary extract, or by prostaglandins (natural hormones that make the uterine muscles relax). In the first method, synthetic oxytocin is injected into a vein via a drip. In the second, prostaglandins are introduced in the form of vaginal pessaries. Some obstetricians explain the process in detail to the mother-to-be, and then give her the pessaries to insert at home, usually at around 6am, after which she goes into hospital at a prearranged time, say around 1 or 2pm, following the pattern of a non-induced labour.

Babies may be induced in order to suit hospital timetables, but there are two types of medical reasons for a baby to be born in advance of natural labour.

Baby reasons When the pregnancy has progressed well but the baby is not growing. This means that the placenta is not providing adequate nourishment and, even though the baby will be born underweight, it would do better in the hospital's nursery than waiting for the mother to give birth.

In multiple pregnancies, that is, if you are expecting twins or more, the placenta may sometimes not keep up with feeding and so an induced birth becomes advisable. Multiple births should always take place in hospital, and the delivery should be supervized by an obstetrician.

Mother reasons   If the mother is very short or small-framed, and particularly if her partner happens to be tall, once the baby has reached 5 or 6 lbs (which can be accurately measured through ultrasound (see page 119), the obstetrician is likely to suggest induction. Because of her small size, her birth canal and pelvis will be very shallow and, if the baby gets too big, she would be likely to have an obstructed labor and/or a Caesarean section.

The baby will be constantly monitored, and induction or Caesarian section discussed if you have any of the following conditions: rhesus blood group incompatibility; high blood pressure; heart or kidney disease; diabetes; history of previous stillbirths.

After the birth

No doubt you will have seen beautiful pictures of newborn babies. It can also be helpful before you yourself give birth to see a colour film of the birth of a baby. From this you will realize that birth is accompanied by a lot of fluid and mess, and is not the immaculate affair that many mothers may imagine. Babies are born covered with a white creamy mixture intermixed with bloody fluid from the placenta. However, once the baby is cleaned up, although remaining red and wrinkled for about a week, he or she does become a presentable human being.

Bonding and family relationships   It is important that you hold your baby as quickly as possible after delivery. In most hospitals today, the baby is put immediately onto the mother's stomach and she is encouraged to cuddle her child. This moment of bonding is essential. Something called 'species recognition' also takes place in these crucial first moments after birth — a mother will inspect her newborn child instinctively, to make sure it has all the bits that make it recognizably human. All primates do this. However, different cultural practices vary this process slightly. For Hindus, for instance, it is an insult to be handed an uncleaned baby, particularly a male child, so the baby is washed and swaddled *before* being presented to the mother. You, as the mother, should discuss your preferences and cultural and ethnic practices with your midwife before going into hospital, to ensure that your traditions and wishes are respected. These are important moments for mother and child, and it would be a pity to mar them through preventable misunderstanding.

Even mothers who have never held a baby before learn to recognize their own child's cry within about 48 hours, and within three to four days most mothers and babies will comfortably fall asleep together, fitting neatly into each other's bodies. Most primates hold their babies on the left side, because the rhythmic beating of the mother's heart is comforting to the baby.

The importance of bonding becomes very clear when we consider those families which practise both physical and psychological child battering. It is almost as if the parent has no attachment and wishes to destroy the child she or he does not recognize. In gorillas a dominant male will often pursue a mother and child for mating. However, he will kill the baby before mating with the female, thus ensuring the dominance of his genes in the group. This is analogous to the child battering or even murder that can take place when a mother takes into the house a man who is not her children's father. This is more common than we like to believe. Research studies tell us that the three main causes of child battering and infanticide are alcohol, poverty, and what sociologists term a threat to 'the male prerogative', that is, the man cannot have sex with the woman because the baby is 'in the way'.

Despite the vital importance of bonding, it is equally important as the child develops to realize that you have given birth to a separate individual with his

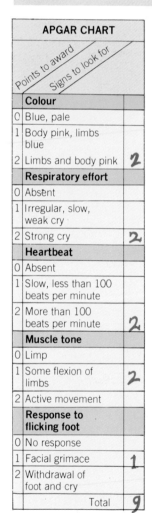

APGAR CHART		
Points to award / Signs to look for		
Colour		
0	Blue, pale	
1	Body pink, limbs blue	
2	Limbs and body pink	2
Respiratory effort		
0	Absent	
1	Irregular, slow, weak cry	
2	Strong cry	2
Heartbeat		
0	Absent	
1	Slow, less than 100 beats per minute	
2	More than 100 beats per minute	2
Muscle tone		
0	Limp	
1	Some flexion of limbs	2
2	Active movement	
Response to flicking foot		
0	No response	
1	Facial grimace	1
2	Withdrawal of foot and cry	
	Total	9

The Apgar scale *is an assessment by medical staff of the baby's condition at birth. The five tests are done again within a few minutes and most babies score nine or ten by then.*

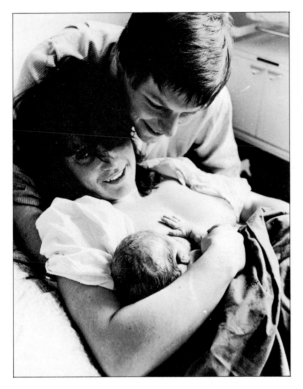

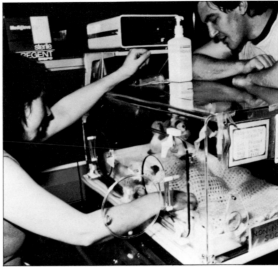

The bonding process takes place most effectively if mother and baby have unrestricted access to each other. Even if the baby is in the special care unit she will respond in many ways to the special sound of your voice and you will learn to distinguish her various gurgles and cries. Staff in the unit will encourage you to help with feeding and care.

or her own personality and destiny. The child's individuality must be respected, just as your needs must be recognized and respected, if he or she is to develop successfully into an adult capable of going out into the world.

Special care units

With the first baby it is quite normal to feel anxious when you cannot see, smell, or touch him or her. If for some reason your baby has to go into a special care baby unit it is therefore essential for you both that you spend as much time there as possible. Even tiny babies with breathing difficulties can be aware of a mother's touch and a mother's voice, and the essential bonding process can take place.

These units care for babies who, because they are small or because they are sick, need high technology medicine. The modern statistics coming out of these units indicate that, except in the case of severe congenital defects, the chances for the baby are excellent.

Feeding your baby

Breast-feeding One of the first signs that you are pregnant is a pricking sensation around the nipples, even before you have missed a period. And throughout the entire pregnancy your breasts will grow and sometimes leak fluid, which may be stimulated involuntarily every time you see or pick up a baby. In this way you are made aware of the potential of breast feeding long before your body is ready for the experience.

Somewhere around mid-pregnancy it is sensible to start treating the nipples and the areolae with surgical spirit to harden up the skin and prevent later chapping or irritation from the baby's sucking. After delivery, it usually takes from a few hours to a couple of days for the milk to 'come down'. (So do not worry that you cannot satisfactorily nourish your baby, if there is this initial delay.) A fatty substance called colostrum is the first sign of this milk supply.

Two things are important:
- Your body must learn to give up its milk.
- The baby must learn to suck.

At this time, you need to drink a lot of fluids, to be comfortable, calm and relaxed, and to have a lot of patience. Many babies start off very

129

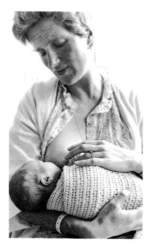

Breast milk is usually the perfect food for human babies.

The best way to ensure a successful start to breast-feeding is to put the baby to the breast as soon as possible after delivery. Once lactation (breast-feeding) is established, you will find it both pleasurable and convenient. In the first four weeks of life two hourly feeding is about right. The once-advocated four hour schedule does not suit many babies.

enthusiastically, taking great big gulps and then, feeling full and tired, will go to sleep on you before having taken enough. To keep your baby awake, talk or sing to him or her (not lullabies!) and if necessary gently pinch the baby's toes. Another trick is to lick and gently blow on the forehead, because a sense of freshness keeps a baby awake. You may receive a few looks of surprise from your newborn, but persevere.

Breast-feeding can be a source of great sensual delight for both you and your baby. Furthermore, it is often much easier when you are travelling or are away from home to breast feed rather than to prepare a bottle. But breast and bottle feeding are not mutually exclusive. There is no truth in the old wives' tale that babies find it easier to suck from a bottle than a breast, and many working mothers can continue an evening breast-feed until the baby is a year old or more, to their mutual pleasure.

Bottle feeding For all sorts of reasons, some women find they cannot or do not want to breast feed their babies. In no way should they be made to feel guilty or concerned about this. Their babies will thrive on bottle milk, so long of course as it is always made up exactly as directed. (*Never* add 'a little more formula' in the mistaken belief that it will be even better for your baby. It will *not*.) So many of us now have become entranced by the back-to-the-earth image of the blissful mother breast feeding her hungry baby that when — for whatever reason — we don't quite fit the picture, we may become anxious and depressed, feeling ourselves to be inadequate and fearful that our babies will not thrive. This does nothing to help the relationship between mother and baby, and the blow to her self-esteem may aggravate possible post-natal depression, making the experience of having a new baby a negative rather than a happy one.

One of the positive aspects of bottle feeding, is the fact that fathers can help more, giving them a sense of involvement and giving the mothers either more sleep or more time off. What is essential during either kind of feeding is that both the person giving sustenance and the baby have enough time and privacy to enjoy the experience.

Babies learn eye-to-eye contact during feeding, and in the good manners and mutual respect learnt during the first year of life, particularly in the establishing of dependable feeding patterns, lie a sound foundation for the 'Terrible Twos' when, unless you both trust each other, mealtimes can be a battleground. It is thus important to allow these early feeds plenty of time in order to establish the proper socialization of mealtimes.

Caring for yourself

Although your baby has now left your body, for the next 20 years you will be rather 'a hostage of fortune'. Giving birth and becoming a successful mother actually change your body and your personality. There are women, for instance, who may have spent the last ten years of their lives in a competitive work environment who, once they become mothers, are made very much aware of the value of human life and have a greatly enhanced response to other people, to animals and even to plants.

Even if your full-time energies have not been directed outside the home, in the shape of a career, you will find that your priorities change radically once you have a baby. A woman's relationship with the baby's father changes greatly; whereas before the birth many marriages revolve around the daily habit of a woman looking after a man, once there is a baby in the house, most men realize that they now have to share with their child the caring affection that they previously enjoyed alone.

Depending on the character of your baby — and some babies require a great deal more attention than others — you will find you have less and less time for yourself and your own interests. It is most important, therefore, for you to accept all offers of help, particularly from your partner, as it is much better in the long run for both of you not to feel that *you* are the only person who can care for the baby. Sharing responsibility for the care of your baby will enrich the relationship between all three of you.

In the first few days after giving birth you may well be assailed by very mixed emotions. You will have the pride and joy of holding your baby son or daughter in your arms at last … instead of carrying around an anonymous lump in your abdomen, given to kicking vigorously from time to time. But your baby will be making his or her presence apparent in other, demanding ways — crying being the principal one.

Also, if you are in a busy ward, surrounded by other mothers with babies, the noise may be considerable just when you most want to rest quietly and recover from the intense physical and emotional experience of giving birth. Console yourself with the thought that all the other mothers are feeling much the same: at one moment almost euphoric with happiness and the next quite the opposite. Particularly if you are usually of a very even temperament you may wonder — why do I feel like this, and will I ever feel self-confident again? Be reassured. These feelings are perfectly natural and it is only a temporary phase brought about by a massive adjustment in your hormonal balance. Try to stay as relaxed as possible and if you have any worries, either about your baby or yourself, don't be diffident about discussing them with your midwife. And whenever quiet moments do occur during the day, take a cat-nap.

Stitches If you have had an episiotomy (see page 126), and the stitches cause some soreness, bathing the area with warm water containing a generous handful of salt will help. Some hospitals will supply salt for this purpose; if yours does not, ask one of your visitors to bring in some. Always take care to dry the area thoroughly, but gently, afterwards. You will probably be supplied with a rubber ring to ease discomfort when you sit up – and if not, do ask for one. If the discomfort is considerable, ask for pain-killing tablets.

You may also find it difficult to control passing water or opening your bowels, or, because soreness can be aggravated by these important functions you may try to avoid doing either. Again, do discuss either problem with your midwife. She will be able to help. You can also help yourself by eating as much as you can of vegetables, salads and fresh fruit. Stitches of this kind usually simply dissolve in about a week, by which time the tear or cut will have healed.

Piles These, too, can be a temporary problem after delivery. They are caused by all the pushing you needed to do while in labour. Again, a rubber ring will make sitting more comfortable and the diet suggested above should make moving your bowels easier.

Bleeding It is normal to lose blood, sometimes in large clots, from your vagina for a few days after the birth, and you will probably also experience contractions of your womb (uterus). This is all perfectly natural at this stage — your womb is expelling blood and debris so that it can return to its pre-pregnancy state. Contractions may be particularly noticeable if you are breast-feeding your baby, because the act of suckling stimulates the contractions and aids the womb's speedy return to pre-birth size.

When you first get out of bed, take it slowly, because you are bound to feel a bit shaky and uncertain to begin with. Start by gently swinging your legs over the side of the bed and, in a sitting position, swing each leg in turn gently backwards and forwards a few times. This will prevent a 'pins and needles' sensation in your feet when you first stand on them. Then gently draw in your pelvic muscles as best you can and try to keep them drawn in and up until you are really steady on your feet. It is quite usual to experience a slight dropping sensation inside at this point, and it can be disconcerting if you're not expecting it. But, in fact, it is a normal reaction and will pass. Your body will soon be restored to normal and you will have control of those muscles once

Some temporary discomforts

Getting up

131

again if you practise post-natal exercises regularly — but don't do these too energetically to begin with.

Going home

If there are no complications, your hospital stay may be only a matter of days but, before you leave, do discuss with your midwife any doubts — however small they may seem — regarding caring for your baby, or yourself. For some time you will receive regular home visits, but the more informed and satisfied you are at the outset, the more confident you will feel. Below are a few of the subjects you may want to clarify.

Contraception and sex It is a good idea to discuss the form of contraception most suitable for you in the first few weeks or months after birth. It is clearly not possible to give advice here, because much will depend on your personal situation. But, certainly, your midwife or doctor can give helpful guidance. Try to discuss this very important topic when your partner can be present too. If it is then recommended that he should use a sheath when, previously, you have always been responsible for contraception, he will know why this is advisable. How long you should wait before resuming full sexual activity will again

POST-NATAL EXERCISES

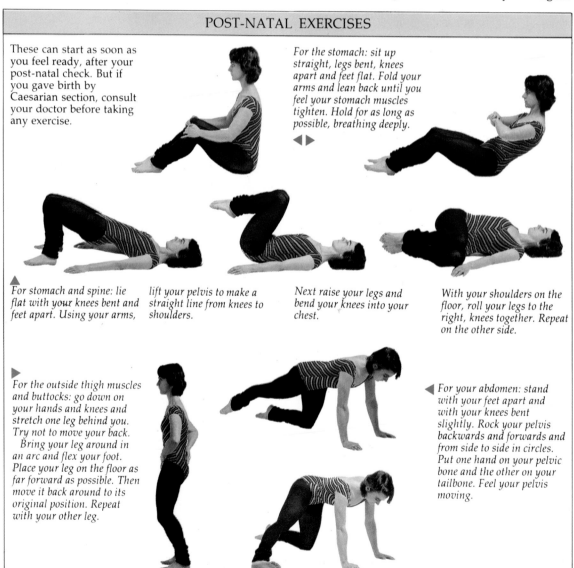

These can start as soon as you feel ready, after your post-natal check. But if you gave birth by Caesarian section, consult your doctor before taking any exercise.

For the stomach: sit up straight, legs bent, knees apart and feet flat. Fold your arms and lean back until you feel your stomach muscles tighten. Hold for as long as possible, breathing deeply.

For stomach and spine: lie flat with your knees bent and feet apart. Using your arms,

lift your pelvis to make a straight line from knees to shoulders.

Next raise your legs and bend your knees into your chest.

With your shoulders on the floor, roll your legs to the right, knees together. Repeat on the other side.

For the outside thigh muscles and buttocks: go down on your hands and knees and stretch one leg behind you. Try not to move your back.
  Bring your leg around in an arc and flex your foot. Place your leg on the floor as far forward as possible. Then move it back around to its original position. Repeat with your other leg.

For your abdomen: stand with your feet apart and with your knees bent slightly. Rock your pelvis backwards and forwards and from side to side in circles. Put one hand on your pelvic bone and the other on your tailbone. Feel your pelvis moving.

depend on such factors as your physical condition, so do ask for guidance if you are in any doubt about this.

Rhesus negative mothers If you are a rhesus negative mother with a rhesus positive partner, it is usual for you to be offered an injection within three days of the birth, to protect your next baby against anaemia. If no-one mentions this within the first day or two, raise the matter with your midwife.

Rubella This is the best time also to have immunization against rubella (German measles), if you were not immune during your pregnancy. Any future babies you may wish to have will then be protected. Be careful not to become pregnant again for at least three months after immunization.

Post-natal depression

The fatigue that you encounter in the first weeks following birth is due to changes in your hormonal state following delivery of the placenta. Most mothers shed a tear or two and experience a feeling of anti-climax at this time. But about one-fifth of all mothers experience real post-natal depression which is serious, profound and can last up to a year. In some rare cases — in a condition known as puerperal psychosis — the woman may lose all grip on reality and there is a real danger that she may injure her baby or commit suicide or infanticide.

Women who are accustomed to experiencing moderate to severe pre-menstrual tension will recognize the feelings that they may encounter — wild crying fits, angry screaming spells and carbohydrate cramming. Other symptoms are feeling worthless and unable to cope, hating the baby, feeling anxious for its safety and their own sanity, and any other symptoms associated with pre-menstrual tension. Post-natal depression results from a similar hormone imbalance.

The partner, friends and relatives of a woman undergoing such depression should try to be as understanding and supportive as possible:
● They should avoid making the mother feel guilty, and allow her to express her feelings of anxiety and fear.
● They should avoid pointing out shortcomings relating to her appearance, her home and so on.
● They should avoid suggesting she is being lazy if she is sleeping a lot — she probably needs all the sleep she can get at this time.

Her partner may also be feeling anxious, guilty, puzzled and — eventually — resentful; remarks like 'Why is she doing this to me?' are common. Fathers may well need as much support as mothers in the first months after the birth.

It must be emphasized that postnatal depression of this type is an illness and professional help must be sought from a social worker or doctor. Contacting a self-help group (details page 142), to draw strength and reassurance from other women who have experienced similar depressions is a very positive step and may well pave the way to recovery.

The first weeks at home

Once you are back in the familiar surroundings of your own home you will soon establish a routine that is best for you. But remember, even if you are feeling fully recovered, you do need rest periods for a while. Fortunately, many employers now allow new fathers a few days leave in which to help out. If that is the case for you, take full advantage of this assistance, particularly with chores that involve lifting, or carrying heavy weights (such as shopping), or very energetic movement. If he is not used to helping, chores may not be done quite so efficiently to begin with, but he will learn with practice and, in the meantime, if the house looks less than perfectly organized — well, that is nothing to worry about.

Post-natal check-up Even if you are feeling fine, it is a sensible precaution to have a medical check-up about six weeks after the birth, and this may well be organized as a matter of routine by the hospital. If not, it can be carried out by your doctor. This is a good opportunity for you to raise any questions you may have. Also, if you are still having a vaginal discharge or any physical discomfort, it can be checked out and any necessary treatment provided.

- A urine test will be done to check that your kidneys are functioning properly.
- Your blood pressure will be checked.
- You will be weighed to check that you have lost most, or all of the additional weight put on in pregnancy.
- An internal examination will confirm that your womb (uterus) is back to its pre-pregnancy size and the pelvic muscles are returning to normal.
- You may also have a cervical smear test. It is a good idea to have one of these anyway.

Even if you believe that your general health is good, it is no bad thing to have this confirmed by a medical practitioner.

Miscarriage

One of the outcomes you are likely to experience, once you have decided that you are pregnant, is early pregnancy failure — or, in ordinary language, a miscarriage. This may sound startling but statistics suggest that 85 per cent of fertilized eggs do not give rise to a living baby. That is, only 15 per cent go through to full term. Some of these lost babies have in fact never been more than what is termed a 'blighted ovum' — that is, true fertilization has not taken place. Although the uterus has responded as though there is a normal pregnancy, the amniotic sac is empty; within a few weeks bleeding occurs and the pregnancy test thereafter becomes negative. But for more than 80 per cent of all cases of women who do experience a miscarriage, no identifiable cause is ever found.

In a study involving nurses who wished to become pregnant it was found that in the majority of those who had a very early positive pregnancy test the pregnancy nevertheless failed. In fact, the percentage of women — around 20 or 25 per cent — whose pregnancy continued to full term was exactly the same as the success rate in an established artificial insemination or test-tube baby programme. Many of us must therefore experience multiple early pregnancy failure without ever realizing that we have had a miscarriage. Until about 30 days after fertilization the amount of tissue involved is so minute that we just think we have had a delayed period. However, after the second missed period, which is somewhere between six and eight weeks of pregnancy, most women realize then when bleeding occurs that they are having a miscarriage.

The woman who has embarked on a pregnancy with the happy anticipation of motherhood will feel deeply deprived and will grieve for this unknown baby; it is not wise for her to begin another pregnancy until she has worked through her grief and come to terms with it. Each woman is different and her mind and body may be ready to attempt another pregnancy within six weeks or six months. Doctors, if asked, will most often say 'Wait six months', and what is essential is for those parents to make a careful analysis of their diet and their life in general and then to decide when to embark on another pregnancy with the aid of good preconceptual care. Physiologically, there are various tests that can be carried out to tell you when your body has started ovulating again, and although such tests are extremely rarely performed in Britain, it might perhaps be a good idea, particularly for women in their late thirties, to ask a doctor about the possibilities.

Stillbirth

A baby is said to be stillborn if it is born dead any time after 28 weeks of pregnancy.

Stillbirths fall into two categories: those which are expected, and those which occur unexpectedly during labour. Factors which influence the first category include such things as retro-placental haemorrage (a leak of blood behind the placental vessels inside the uterine wall); the mother being diabetic

THE THREE MAIN CAUSES OF MISCARRIAGE

ALCOHOL AND SEX

An analysis of the predisposing factors for a miscarriage to occur suggests that even moderate alcohol intake, if associated with sex, can cause bleeding in pregnancy. But alcohol, even without sex, cannot actively do good either to mother or child. Previous generations of women have always assumed that it was unwise to have sex during pregnancy. Now, many physicians advise patients to continue sexual activity as long as they feel comfortable. But although contraceptive devices might at this stage seem to be rather superfluous, many doctors think that sex without is unwise and that a barrier method, such as a diaphragm or a sheath, is a sensible precaution. (The pill and the IUD must *not* be used at this time.) As always, the choice to have sex must be mutual. Many women lose interest in sex during pregnancy; any woman who has this reaction should trust this instinctual response and resist the persuasion of the latest sex manuals or an importunate lover.

SERIOUS DISEASE

Diabetes   Advances in medical technology and a greater understanding of metabolic differences between diabetics and non-diabetics have meant that women with diabetes can now give birth to healthy, normal babies. As recently as the 1950s this was not so; regulation of the flow of blood sugar and insulin through the mother's placenta to the fetus was a hit-and-miss business and many of the babies died either in the birth process or shortly after from respiratory diseases. Now diabetic women can plan a pregnancy with much greater confidence. Special units exist which teach them how to monitor their own blood sugar, and during pregnancy and labor the right metabolic balance of sugar and insulin is maintained so that the baby develops normally, without diabetes.

Acute viral illnesses   During the early stage of pregnancy the growing fetus and its placental attachment are particularly vulnerable, and, although the hazards of specific viruses such as rubella (German measles) have been clearly documented during the last two decades, the detection of other viral illnesses such as flu and acute fever is extremely difficult. Any period of feverish illness in early pregnancy should be investigated immediately; mother and baby are seriously at risk.

Obesity   The most common type of malnutrition in the Western world is generalized obesity. This often increases during the first pregnancy as, somewhat unfairly, women who are already overweight tend to gain much more weight than those who start off reasonably slim. Recent studies show that there is also a significant increase in raised blood pressure and it has been found that the loss of babies is more than double that of women with normal weight.

Like all metabolic disorders, the effect of obesity is more severe in women who are aged 35 and over than in those still in their twenties, because after 35 the whole body metabolism tends to slow down. This can, however, be countered through proper nutrition and exercise, particularly in the preconceptual and antenatal period, but also as part of a healthy way of life (see the chapter on Health Cultivation).

Heart disease and kidney disease   The two other conditions which can seriously affect the well-being and life expectancy of the fetus and mother in early pregnancy are heart disease and kidney disease. Again, women with either of these medical problems should register with a high-risk unit, preferably before they are pregnant, because even women who have had kidney transplants can now successfully give birth to a normal baby.

GENETIC CAUSES

The figures show that more than half of all early miscarriages occur because of an abnormality of the embryo. If the sperm and egg are not both carrying 23xx or xy chromosomes then the embryo will be defective; in many cases a spontaneous early miscarriage will take place.

or having some disease causing lack of oxygen or nourishment to the baby; and, very rarely these days, rhesus problems.

Understanding obstetricians and helpful midwives can be of the greatest assistance in helping the mother understand the process and so be prepared for an adequate working out of her grief. The parents of an expected stillborn baby have usually overcome the shock of knowing the baby had died before birth, and are therefore prepared for the final chapter when all hope is lost and the mother gives birth to a dead baby.

The second category of still birth is due to an accident in labour — a sudden haemorrage between the placenta and the uterine wall, for example, or the umbilical cord becoming twisted around the baby's neck.

Such an experience is not only a dreadful event for the parents, but is also profoundly shocking for all concerned with the delivery. The whole delivery unit will experience some degree of grief. Until recently many obstetricians were totally unable to deal with their own sense of failure. They could not communicate with the grieving mother, and usually delegated any discussion to a junior doctor or the nursing staff. Many women have described in detail how they were cruelly kept in the same ward as mothers nursing their babies, and how this prevented their own understanding of their grief.

Nowadays in most maternity units obstetric staff will understand enough about their own reactions to give proper care and counselling. Allowing the parents to hold the dead baby and perhaps to keep a photograph of the child have been found to be a great help in the acceptance of the loss of the baby and their working through of grief.

Situations in which a baby is born with a birth defect can result in similar difficulties; the best help for grieving mothers may come from others who have undergone the experience, rather than from health care professionals.

Abortion

In lay terms we tend to use the word 'abortion' for a pregnancy terminated upon the mother's request or because a medical diagnosis of a birth defect has been made. In terms of the social effects of abortion, the majority of women who choose a legal termination of an unwanted pregnancy do not experience as much long-term grief, guilt and distress as mothers who have had to have a termination because of congenital defects such as Mongolism (Down's syndrome). In an ideal world women would all be clear-headed enough to know when we are having sex for pleasure and when we are having sex in order to get pregnant, and so more than 90 per cent of social abortions could be prevented.

If you have taken a risk and realize that your chances of conception are quite high, it is useful to consider the morning-after pill, see page 31 on post coital contraception. If your period is late and you think that you might be pregnant, one of the most infallible ways to find out is to have a blood test for traces of what is called a beta HCG, which is one of the sub-units of the pregnancy hormone, human chorionic gonadotrophin. There are, however, other pregnancy tests more readily available (see page 112). The risks of any woman undergoing an abortion are twofold:

The surgical risks of anaesthesia   In many countries a large proportion of terminations of pregnancy are performed under a local anaesthetic with little or no risk to the patient's brain. In Britain, where the newer techniques using day care and local anaesthesia are not widely available, any woman has to consider the faint possibility that she may die or be seriously brain damaged by general anaesthesia.

The surgical risks of infection or haemorrhage   The actual surgical part of an abortion is very much less dangerous than the risks from anaesthesia. The risks of incurring negative surgical consequences after an abortion in terms of problems such as infection, haemorrhage leading to chronic pelvic pain, obstetric incompetence, damage to childbearing capacity or reduction in sexual happiness, are less than 8 per cent.

However, 92 per cent of abortions *are* successful and have no side effects, while maternal deaths from childbirth, although rare in the Western world, do still occur.

Some women *have* to consider abortion in lieu of long-term contraception for a variety of reasons, and for these women — indeed for any woman who considers terminating a pregnancy — early diagnosis and procedures will greatly reduce any possible negative side effects, both physical and psychological. If a pregnancy is terminated very early, before the woman's body has become fully 'programmed' to being a mother — that is, before the hormones which produce the nesting instinct and all that this entails have got fully into gear — the feelings of grief, regret, guilt, horror or failure that many women report experiencing after an abortion are likely to be less severe. Most women must, however, expect to suffer from some form of depression after an abortion. The woman who claims to feel nothing after terminating a pregnancy is very rare indeed.

Menstrual extraction   If you feel pregnant, or if your period is just one day late, your chances of having an ordinary miscarriage — that is, early pregnancy failure — are about 50 per cent. However, if although you want the pregnancy to terminate you are not willing to take that risk and prefer to wait — if, moreover, you live in the right area and are prepared to defend the legality of the operation — menstrual extraction can be performed under local anaesthesia. It involves between three and five minutes of discomfort but there is virtually nothing by way of side effects. Whether or not this procedure

Methods of abortion early in pregnancy

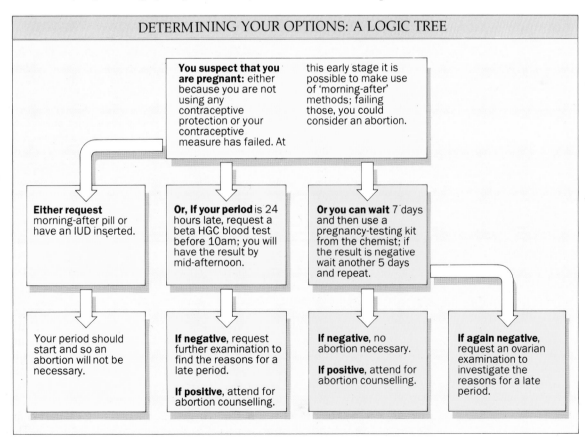

DETERMINING YOUR OPTIONS: A LOGIC TREE

You suspect that you are pregnant: either because you are not using any contraceptive protection or your contraceptive measure has failed. At this early stage it is possible to make use of 'morning-after' methods; failing those, you could consider an abortion.

Either request morning-after pill or have an IUD inserted.

Or, if your period is 24 hours late, request a beta HGC blood test before 10am; you will have the result by mid-afternoon.

Or you can wait 7 days and then use a pregnancy-testing kit from the chemist; if the result is negative wait another 5 days and repeat.

Your period should start and so an abortion will not be necessary.

If negative, request further examination to find the reasons for a late period.

If positive, attend for abortion counselling.

If negative, no abortion necessary.

If positive, attend for abortion counselling.

If again negative, request an ovarian examination to investigate the reasons for a late period.

Vacuum suction is the accepted method for terminating a pregnancy before ten weeks. It is usually performed on an out-patient basis. You will probably experience painful cramps but you should have fully recovered in a few days.

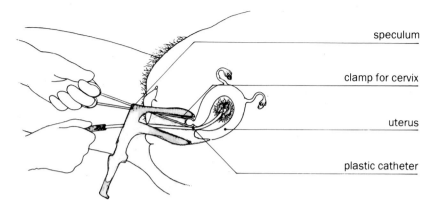

speculum

clamp for cervix

uterus

plastic catheter

is successful depends largely on the training and experience of the team performing the extraction.

Between four and ten weeks, the contents of the uterus can be removed in exactly the same way by vacuum suction after dilating the cervical os. This takes between 10 and 15 minutes and can be done under either local or general anaesthesia. Indeed, for any woman who has already had a baby, a gentle and proficient operator can perform the operation with a plastic cannula, without using any anaesthesia.

Dilatation and curettage (D&C) Most D&Cs are done under a general anaesthetic and, as a result, have a higher incidence of backache, possibly due to the old-fashioned, weighted speculum which is used .

Methods of abortion after ten weeks

Induction After ten weeks of pregnancy all side effects are greatly increased. And whereas a very experienced operator can evacuate the uterus up to 18 weeks by similar methods of dilatation and curettage, it is very distressing for everybody concerned. In most large units where late terminations are performed (usually for strictly medical reasons), therefore, the induction of early labour by putting prostaglandin or saline into the uterus is much preferred. At the same time the medical team may feel it is necessary to open the cervix with either prostaglandin pessaries or laminaria suppositories.

Hystereotomy As a last resort, a patient who has decided upon sterilization can sometimes have a safe, late abortion by mini-Caesarian section. However, the side effects are statistically increased and most gynaecologists prefer that these procedures be kept quite separate, as there is the risk that a woman who chooses to be sterilized while her emotions are stirred by an unwanted pregnancy may bitterly regret it later. There is also the possibility that tied tubes will re-canalize (open up again), leading to a vastly increased risk of unwanted pregnancy.

Abortion counselling

Most of the major abortion units have trained counsellors who can greatly assist you in taking the decision as to whether or not to terminate a pregnancy. Much mileage has been derived from the present situation in which a woman who refuses to maintain her pregnancy is given a lot of counselling whereas a woman who chooses motherhood may be pushed by on the conveyor belt system of modern maternity and antenatal care with very little help to understand and cope with her ambivalent feelings. In my experience, fewer than 2 per cent of women, having decided upon abortion, need any form of counselling except regarding the risks for the individual woman at the particular stage of pregnancy at which she presents. (Paradoxically, one of the leading exponents of early abortion in this country, Dr Peter Huntingford, feels that as the physical risk of early abortion is much less than the physical risks of childbirth at full term, all women can be considered to be acting in their own best interests if they choose to have an early abortion!)

Infertility

Until quite recently infertility or inability to give birth to living children was a taboo subject. The facts are that somewhere between 15 and 20 per cent of couples have difficulties in achieving conception. Infertility is no longer considered to be shameful, and with the recent well-publicized, spectacular successes of the new technologies of fertilization, the treatment of infertility has become an exciting and expanding field of modern medicine.

Infertility used to be considered in some way a woman's 'fault'; it was always she who was said to be barren. But recent statistics show that in couples in their thirties around 50 per cent of infertility is due to an inadequate supply of living sperm. So any couple considering a consultation regarding their inability to start a family should begin by getting a total sperm count and analysis. This can be done quite cheaply by any reputable medical laboratory if you prefer to get a quick analysis rather than go through the lengthy and costly procedure of consultation and referral. However, beware the self-styled infertility analysts advertising in the press who charge grossly inflated prices for this simple service.

Infertility tests are not generally carried out by doctors. But they will refer you, if necessary, to a specialist. The Family Planning Service, which is part of the National Health Service, has recently become more interested in actually planning pregnancies as opposed to preventing them, and most now offer early fertility tests.

If you are under 30, have been trying for twelve months and are still not pregnant, it is sensible to have two non-invasive tests done: firstly, the sperm count mentioned above and, secondly, the woman should have a pelvic examination carried out by a gynaecologist. If the sperm count is normal and the pelvic examination shows nothing amiss, the next step is to use a menstrual diary (see page 12) and continue trying for another four to six cycles. Sometimes, just by giving up smoking and alcohol many couples achieve the much-wanted pregnancy.

If, however, at the end of this time you still have not succeeded in becoming pregnant, it is sensible for your partner to have a repeat sperm count with added tests for sperm mobility and sperm antibodies, and for you to have ultrasound evaluation of ovulation. If these tests are normal and you still do not conceive within one year of planning a pregnancy, take your problem to an infertility specialist who will advise on further tests.

If you are aged over 30 you need to take special care regarding your eating, drinking and smoking habits. If necessary, seek specialist preconceptual advice and care. And do not wait for more than three menstrual cycles before undergoing the initial infertility tests outlined above.

The new conceptions

Since the birth in 1978 of the first test-tube baby, Louise Brown, every aspect of both the medical and the ethical problems of the new conceptions have been debated in medical circles at great lengths.

It is important to remember that each baby that is born, regardless of its origin, is an individual under the UNESCO charter of rights devised for all the world's children. A potential human being exists from about 40 days after conception. In the light of this, every adult who is concerned with the birth of this potential child, from the mother-to-be or the gynaecologist who is making every effort to find out if this will be a healthy baby, to the scientist in a laboratory, every adult involved in producing a test-tube baby, must have the same moral attitude to this baby as they would have towards any other.

Doctors, by virtue of their intimate knowledge of their patients, are sometimes asked to decide which women have the potential to be a competent surrogate mother, see page 140. It is irrational to assume, as detractors sometimes do, that because a surrogate is being paid, her motives are not of the highest. Just as an obstetrician will share in the joy of the parents in welcoming a healthy baby into the world, so the surrogate mother may share in the joy that she brings to the infertile couple.

Certainly she will be far more actively involved than the many healthy medical students who sell their sperm for AID (artificial insemination by donor male) with no emotion and no intellectual curiosity for the babies they have fathered.

Artificial insemination by husband (AIH)

This is a method used when the man has a low count of healthy sperm or if he consistently ejaculates prematurely. The sperm is placed gently and carefully inside the cervix, overcoming any potential problem it encounters with hostile mucus and considerably reducing the time the sperm takes to reach the fallopian tubes for fertilization to take place. This process has become much easier and more efficient, thanks to accurate monitoring of ovulation by ultrasound techniques.

For couples who find this method too impersonal, however, there is an alternative. They can be taught how to use a simple cap device to which is attached a thin rubber tube. The woman simply inserts the cap over the neck of her womb and the husband then injects his own collected sperm through the tube with the aid of a syringe. The cap is left in place overnight in the hope that some of the sperm will reach the uterus. AIH can also be used in combination with freezing techniques, particularly useful when a man is being treated for cancer with chemotherapy which seriously impairs sperm production.

Artificial insemination by donor (AID)

If AIH proves unsuccessful after several attempts, but the husband does have some sperm, AID using donated sperm with the husband's sample may be tried. This means that the resulting pregnancy has *some* chance of being his.

Or, if the husband has no sperm at all, or is a known carrier of certain hereditary disorders, AID solely by an anonymous donor may be considered.

All men who serve as donors are very carefully screened to ensure that they are physically fit — and attempts are made to match both physical and intellectual characteristics with those of the male partner. The freezing of sperms has been a useful development in this process.

The donor has no knowledge of the couple to whom his sperm will be given and most couples simply raise the AID baby as their legitimate child — although the legality of putting the male partner's name on the birth certificate is doubted by many lawyers.

In vitro fertilization (IVF)

The first 'test-tube' babies were conceived by taking the woman's own egg, fertilizing it in a small dish in a laboratory, and then replacing it in the woman's uterus. This process is also called embryo transfer (ET).

The technique now has several variations. One method is to implant more than one fertilized egg in the woman's uterus, to increase her chances of producing a full-term, live baby, but it has also created a number of multiple pregnancies. Aside from the subsequent physical risks and difficulties to both mother and baby, the emotional and physical stresses of raising such a family can be somewhat frightening.

In 1978, the obstetrician Patrick Steptoe and reproductive physiologist Dr Robert Edwards achieved the major breakthrough in this technique of 'test-tube' pregnancy. Treating a woman who had been unable to conceive naturally due to blocked fallopian tubes, they removed an egg from her ovary, fertilized it with sperm donated by her husband, grew the egg *in vitro* (in the laboratory) to the eight-to-sixteen-cell stage and then implanted it into her uterus, where it grew to full-term normally. The technique is fraught with difficulties and is still not widely available, but Steptoe and Edwards set up a clinic in Cambridge to continue with this work and they, and other doctors in the UK and abroad, have since achieved similar successes.

One of the problems with test-tube baby techniques has been the high medical costs; these include one or two nights in hospital, expensive hormone evaluation of the mother's serum and the need to collect the eggs with the aid of direct vision through a laparoscope. (This is a tube with a viewing light attached to a needle to remove the eggs from the ovary, and is inserted through the mother's abdomen.)

However, an out-patient technique has now been perfected which makes use of ultrasound. The pictures locate the egg, and a fine needle is inserted into the woman's abdomen, removing the egg without using expensive surgery. This technique can be carried out for a fraction of the earlier cost.

When the Australian freezing methods with multiple implantations are combined with this technique the success rate promises to be much higher than the slight chances that women have at present using IVF on its own. Success rates at the moment vary from 8 per cent to occasionally as high as 20 per cent, but it is claimed that with the freezing of ova the weaker eggs will die, leaving only the strongest for fertilization and implantation.

There has been much publicity in the past year or so for this comparatively new development in assisting childless couples, which has about a 20 per cent success rate. In cases where the source of infertility is traced to the woman and is untreatable, some couples have turned to women willing to bear a child by having the husband's sperm implanted by artificial insemination.

Surrogate motherhood

Surrogate motherhood is also useful in the case of a woman who has had a partial hysterectomy but has retained healthy egg-producing ovaries; it is possible for an egg to be surgically removed and fertilized with her partner's sperm. It is then implanted in the uterus of the surrogate mother who will have received hormone treatment to prepare her uterus for the pregnancy.

After the birth the surrogate mother hands the baby over to the natural father and his partner, having signed documents forgoing all rights to the child. However, one major difficulty in this situation is that there is always the possibility that the surrogate mother may become so attached to the baby that she will not feel able to surrender it to the hopeful parents, thus creating a position of legal complexity and enormous emotional stress for all three.

ADOPTION AND FOSTERING

For couples who decide to adopt, whether because of an infertile relationship or as an extension to their family, the major change in recent years is that tiny babies are no longer readily available for adoption, except for those babies born with a handicap. Improvements in contraceptive methods, availability of legal abortion and the breaking down of the stigma associated with raising a child alone have meant that the majority of children available for adoption are older and those with special needs — either emotional problems or mental or physical handicap.

Whatever your reasons for adoption, you will need to go through an adoption agency in your area — either a local authority department or a voluntary agency which might be affiliated to a church.

Most agencies will expect you to be in a stable relationship and be in good health and they will probably dissuade you from adopting a child from another race. It is now widely felt that children need to share the cultural identity of their families. If you are single, you may be able to persuade an agency to let you adopt, particularly if the child is in need of a one-to-one relationship.

Fostering is different to adoption in that the child will eventually be taken away from you. You can apply for adoption if you have fostered a child for more than five years, but with fostering, your sympathies must also lie with the child's natural parents. Fostering is an excellent option for couples with well-adjusted families where children in need can be offered a stable, happy environment while their natural parents sort out their problems. Some foster parents offer their services in an emergency with only one or two hours' notice.

Whatever your choice, adoption or fostering, you will have the advice and support of the social services and you may qualify for allowances to help you to cope.

Useful addresses

CHAPTER 1
THE SEXUAL WOMAN

Contraception and health care
Family Planning Information Service
27-35 Mortimer Street
London W1 (01) 636 7866

FPA (Northern Ireland)
47 Botanic Avenue
Belfast 7 (0232) 225458

FPA (Scotland)
4 Clifton Street
Glasgow 3 (041) 333 9696

FPA (Wales)
6 Windsor Place
Cardiff (0222) 387471

Irish FPA
15 Mountjoy Square
Dublin 1
Dublin 740723

Physical and sexual harassment
A number of centres exist throughout
Britain which provide support and
temporary refuge to women and
children who are suffering physical,
sexual or mental violence; for details
of your nearest centre contact one of
the following:

Women's Aid Federation
52-54 Featherstone Street
London EC1 (01) 251 6429

Northern Ireland Women's Aid
Federation
143a University Street
Belfast (0232) 249041/249358

Welsh Women's Aid
Incentive House
Adam Street
Cardiff (0222) 388291

Scottish Women's Aid
11 St Colme Street
Edinburgh (031) 225 8011

Incest
A self-help group exists for those
who have suffered incestuous
experiences;

Incest Survivors Group
c/o A Woman's Place
Hungerford House
Victoria Embankment
London WC2

Rape
Rape Crisis Centres now exist in
many cities. The London and
Birmingham centres both have 24
hour lines; contact them for the
telephone number of your nearest
centre.

London Rape Crisis Centre
PO Box 69
London WC1
(01) 278 3956 (office hours)
(01) 837 1600 (24 hour line)

Birmingham Rape Crisis Centre
PO Box 558
Birmingham B3 2HL
(021) 233 2122 (office hours)
(021) 233 2122 (24 hour line)

CHAPTER 2
HEALTH CARE

General information
The Patients Association
Room 33, 18 Charing Cross Road
London WC2 (01) 240 0671
The Patients Association runs an
information service and publishes
Self Help and the Patient – a directory of
organizations concerned with
particular diseases/handicaps.

Community Health Councils
126 Albert Street
London NW1
Your telephone directory will list
your local CHC; each district has one
and they represent 'consumer'
interests in health. Contact them if
you have problems or complaints
about health facilities.

The British Holistic Medical
Association
179 Gloucester Place
London NW1

Chiropractic
British Chiropractic Association
5 First Avenue
Chelmsford, Essex CM1 1RX
The Association keeps a register of
practitioners, and will provide
leaflets and a book list.

Common ailments
DAWN (Drugs Alcohol Women
Nationally)
c/o London Council on Alcoholism
146 Victoria Street London EC4

Alcoholics Anonymous
140a Tatchbrook Street
London, SW1 (01) 834 8202

Anorexic Aid
c/o Alison Cork
The Priory Centre
11 Priory Road
High Wycombe, Bucks

Women's National Cancer Control
Campaign
1 South Audley Street
London W1 (01) 499 7532
The campaign produces material and
visual aids on breast self-examination
and cervical smears. They also offer
help and support to women
undergoing treatment for various
forms of cancer.

Mastectomy Association
26 Harrison Street
London WC1 (01) 837 0908

CHAPTER 3
HEALTH CULTIVATION

Positive health
Health Education Council
78 New Oxford Street
London WC1 (01) 637 1881
The Council organizes campaigns to
increase awareness of positive health
and health matters generally; they
produce a wide range of leaflets and
posters.

CHAPTER 4
THE FERTILE WOMAN

Childbirth
National Childbirth Trust
9 Queensborough Terrace
London W2 (01) 221 3833

Maternity Alliance
309 Kentish Town Road
London NW5 (01) 267 3255
Campaigns for improved services for
pregnant women.

Miscarriage
Miscarriage Association
2 West Vale
Thornhill Road
Dewsbury, W. Yorks WF12 9QH
The Association offers support and
advice to miscarriage sufferers.

Adoption and fostering
British Agencies for Adoption and
Fostering
11 Southwark Street
London SE1 (01) 407 8800

INDEX